"I personally and professionally recommend this book...and have recommended it as a part of a resource guide for the State of Ohio's I Can Cope programs sponsored by the American Cancer Society."

> *Pat Schlosser,* chairman, Service and
> Rehabilitation Committee, Lucas County Unit,
> American Cancer Society

"Provides the cancer patient and family members with a resource when they feel most isolated and know others' help is least likely to be available."

> *Charles Cobau, M.D.,* clinical professor of
> medicine, Medical College of Ohio, Toledo

"Offers proof positive solutions to the catastrophic shock of having cancer."

> *Jean H., R.N.,* a woman who has breast cancer

"Provides 'medicine for the spirit'...the only book I've seen that actively involves the patient as well as the family in emotional healing. It is both simple and powerful."

> *Rita Stoll, R.N.,* oncology nurse

"A valuable tool for working with children who have life-threatening illnesses. We have adopted this book for volunteer training."

> *Rainbow Center,* working with children and
> families with catastrophic illnesses

"My mother has cancer of the pancre[...] book to be very helpful."

> *A family member*

"I love 'The Harbor.'"

> *Mike M.,* a man who has lung cancer

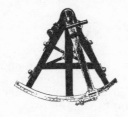

CANCER & HOPE

Charting a Survival Course

Formerly published as *The Cancer Survival Kit*

Judith Garrett Garrison, M.Ed., L.S.W.
Scott Sheperd, Ph.D.

CompCare® Publishers
Minneapolis, Minnesota

Library of Congress Cataloging-in-Publication Data
Garrison, Judith Garrett.
    Cancer and Hope: charting a survival course/Judith Garrett Garrison,
Scott Sheperd.
        p.   cm.
    "Formerly published as The Cancer Survival Kit for cancer patients,
families, and friends."
    Bibliography: p.
    ISBN 0-89638-151-X
    1. Cancer—Psychological aspects. 2. Adjustment (Psychology)
I. Sheperd, Scott, 1945- II. Title.
RC262.G37   1989
155.9'16—dc20   89-7260
                                                                        CIP

Cover design by Jeremy Gale
Interior design by MacLean and Tuminelly

Inquiries, orders, and catalog requests should be
addressed to:
CompCare Publishers
2415 Annapolis Lane
Minneapolis, MN 55441
Call toll free 800/328-3330
(Minnesota residents, 612/559-4800)

5   4   3   2   1
93   92   91   90   89

For people with cancer,
their families, and their friends

Contents

Part Two: The Guide

Part Three: Captain's Log

Part Four: Peace Supplies

Part Five: Your Personal Support Group

Foreword

It is difficult for anyone who has not had cancer to appreciate the emotional challenge the disease poses to cancer patients and their families. The unpredictability of the outcome—and patients' own inability to influence the outcome—make it difficult to mount a positive response. Added to that are the burdens of uncomfortable, prolonged diagnostic and therapeutic procedures, and the loss of dignity associated with the impersonal atmosphere of many hospitals and clinics. Often the busy clinician has insufficient time to address effectively patients' problems in coming to grips emotionally with the diagnosis. Frequently the patient and family members have little guidance as they confront the implications of cancer and learn how to "survive."

How to "survive" emotionally is the subject of *Cancer and Hope: Charting a Survival Course.* For answers, the authors have drawn upon a wealth of personal and professional experience. The book compares the experience of cancer to the voyage of a sailing ship. As the traveler progresses, he or she learns that others have experienced similar feelings about their situation and have successfully completed the same journey.

Since most cancer patients and their families go through this process alone, this book fills an obvious void. It provides the cancer patient and family members with a resource when they feel most isolated and when other help is least likely to be available.

This is the second edition of this book, previously published as *The Cancer Survival Kit.* It offers the same quality of support found by those whose enthusiastic reception of the first edition encouraged this new expanded guide, now called *Cancer and Hope: Charting a Survival Course.*

Charles Cobau, M.D.,
clinical professor of medicine,
Medical College of Ohio, Toledo

A Note from the Authors

Since the first printing of this material as *The Cancer Survival Kit,* we've seen an interesting and wonderful phenomenon: people with illnesses other than cancer have been using the book to help cope with their own emotional turmoil. Their reports reaffirm for us that we were successful in our attempt to write a book about living, hope, courage, support, love, and the belief that we *can* make a difference in our own lives—that a disease can only control our spirits if we let it. Through years of experience we have seen that emotional pain and struggle transcend individual illnesses. Fear is fear, no matter what triggers it. Guilt, depression, and anger are not the private feelings of people with cancer!

Obviously every illness has its own characteristics and we are not medical experts, but we are presenting ideas that we believe are helpful. Readers have confirmed this by telling us how they have used our ideas to cope with AIDS, diabetes, heart disease, and other diseases.

We hope that you or your loved one who may be struggling with a serious illness will find help in *Cancer and Hope: Charting a Survival Course.*

Scott Sheperd
Judith Garrison

Preface

If you are coping with cancer, either personally or as a concerned family member or friend, the goal of this book is to provide you with a means of viewing your illness in a new way. This new perspective will enable you to increase your awareness of yourself and your reactions to situations encountered as you live with cancer. We hope that the information, activities, and images in this book will provide a supportive guide for you as you embark on your journey.

Your journey begins when you receive the diagnosis of cancer. Of course it is a time of apprehension, fear, and uncertainty. The seas are unfamiliar and you are unsure of what you need and what to expect. This book can serve as a chart through these troubled waters, which, though new to you, are not totally uncharted. Many people have made this trip before you, and their experiences shine like beacons to guide new travelers.

Obviously no one can guarantee the physical outcome of cancer. Our goal is to encourage you to play a major, positive role in your journey, both emotionally and spiritually, by making use of the techniques and materials here. We feel that the state of your emotional and spiritual self is as important as that of your physical self and that treating all three equally can contribute significantly to your well-being.

We believe that there is value in looking at your situation symbolically. Images of a traveler experiencing a challenging journey may prompt you to explore more alternatives, avoid some problems and seek innovative solutions to others. The picture of a cancer "victim" facing an incurable disease is a negative image which leaves you stuck in a no-way-out predicament.

We use the theme of a journey by water to parallel the events and situations you might encounter. You focus on the physical, emotional, and spiritual aspects of your journey. And you discover the kinds of sustenance—courage, love, self-esteem, hope—that you will need to survive the trip.

Your journey is not an easy one. It is not one you have chosen for yourself. We hope that as you become more familiar with the seascape you will learn that you have resources available to you, both from without and from within. Using these resources, you will be able to find the courage, faith, and hope to move forward on your course to a place of serenity and acceptance. We also hope that you will see that there can be beauty even in the midst of the difficulties you encounter on your journey through the cancer experience.

Introduction

We realize that in times of depression, illness, and loss, written materials can seem burdensome because of their complexity and bulk. Reading may be difficult due to medications, inability to concentrate, or lack of incentive. Therefore *Cancer and Hope* is designed for easy use. The parts and chapters are intentionally brief and concise. The activities are not complicated or time-consuming.

We have avoided the use of the word "patient" as we feel it implies that everyone living with cancer is perpetually associated with hospitals and doctors' offices. We prefer the image of a person coping with an illness.

Exercises for family and friends are included where appropriate. By "family" we mean anyone who is close to and cares for a person with cancer.

Part One: The Journey

This section equates the experience of cancer with a sea journey—the hazards you may encounter and the points of refuge you will want to seek out. It describes feelings you may have, warning signs of approaching dangers, and ways of avoiding those dangers.

Part Two: The Guide

This guide for a successful journey offers realistic suggestions and activities to be used in response to specific situations you meet along your way.

Part Three: Captain's Log

Here you are encouraged to do one of the most important things a traveler does: record the thoughts and feelings you experience on your journey. A list of questions to ask yourself each day provides a format for your daily entries.

Part Four: Peace Supplies

For times when only the simplest ideas are helpful, this brings you a selection of thoughts and affirmations to steady your course and guide you to your own sense of calm and peace. Choose the thoughts that help you most—and add some of your own.

Part Five: Your Personal Support Group

This section reproduces a dialogue between members of a cancer support group. Since the members are a composite of the many individuals we have worked with, the discussion is real—a typical, honest exchange of ideas and experiences in a group of people who either have cancer or are close to people with cancer.

PART ONE

THE
JOURNEY

Introduction to Part One

You are encouraged to read all of this section, since it can help you with currently troubling situations as it prepares you to avoid future difficulties.

As you chart your voyage, you will find ports and calm waters—like the Island of Magic and the Sea of Serenity. Let these images bring you new ways of perceiving your situation and the encouragement you need to endure. Activities are suggested to guide your use of positive energies.

You will also discover obstacles, like Windless Straits of Boredom and Apathy and Sandbars of Embarrassment and Guilt, each with its own set of warning signs for you to examine. If you find yourself caught in one of these negative emotional places, there is a list of "What to Do"—specifically and generally—to move past them. Some of these ideas for coping with problem areas are especially designed for family members. These "What to Do" suggestions are not exhaustive. Generate your own ideas too. And remember—any of these ideas are only as effective as the strength of your involvement with them. You are the key element!

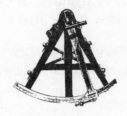

The Ship

The most important part of any journey is the preparation—especially preparing the vehicle in which you will travel. On this particular journey, you are in a unique position; you are not only the captain of the ship but the ship itself. The materials you use and the care you take will define the success of your journey, for your ship must be constructed to endure throughout the trip. Here is a checklist for a successful voyage:

• Your ship must be made of a flexible material to be able to give and take under the shifting pressures of the sea.

• Your ship must not only be resilient, but must be sturdy enough to withstand the many rigors of the trip.

• Your ship must be equipped with a good repair kit for necessary adjustments along the way.

• Your ship must have a good rudder to keep you on your chosen course.

• Your ship must have large sails to catch the winds of motivation.

• Your ship must have a place of comfort and quiet aboard, where you can relax and rest.

• Your ship must have an emergency power source for use when the outside forces fade—when the winds are still.

• Your ship needs a good compass to maintain a strong sense of direction.

• Your ship needs a crow's nest with a telescope, so you can avoid the hazards in your path and look to the heavens for guidance.

• Your ship needs a lantern that will send out a beacon of warmth capable of lighting up the darkest of nights.

• Your ship needs a figurehead with a spirit and character all its own, which gives your craft a spark of life in even the heaviest downpour or the thickest fog.

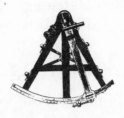

The Harbor of Denial

The Harbor of Denial is a protected inlet mostly surrounded by land which is familiar and comforting. The Harbor of Denial can be a welcome place to stop, especially early in the journey when you're dealing with storms of unwelcome news and waves of shock.

The Harbor of Denial can be a haven of rest, a place to gather strength before returning to the seas better prepared to weather the voyage. Or it can be a place to get stuck. The problem arises when you never leave this harbor, when you pretend that the harbor is the world and don't prepare yourself for the open seas. In fact, you tell yourself that the seas do not exist. You are frightened, but you cannot admit the fear. But there is no way to avoid the seas; the tides draw you to them. You must prepare yourself.

So rest in the Harbor of Denial if you must, but do not linger. Use your time in the harbor to prepare and then activate your inner energy source. And then continue on your journey.

Warning signs of denial are difficult to recognize because the person with the problem, in effect, denies the problem. Your best option is to do the activities included in the "What to Do" section consistently. If you are not misusing denial, the exercises will help you avoid that misuse. If you are denying your problem in a detrimental way, the activities will assist you in moving out of this phase.

Denial: Warning Signs

1. You totally avoid thinking about your physical situation.

2. You refuse to discuss your condition with even those closest to you.

3. You explain away any physical sensations.

4. You seek out quick and easy "cures" for your illness.

5. You refuse to accept medical treatment or change your behaviors into healthier ones because that would mean you are sick and you won't admit that fact.

Denial: What to Do

1. Talk over your fears and concerns with someone you trust. This could be a member of your family, a clergyperson, friend, or counselor. Talking about your feelings will enhance your ability to confront and deal with the issues you face.

2. Think positively about yourself and your ability to cope with the situation. What we tell ourselves often proves to be true. A defeatist attitude can lead to defeat. A progressive, self-help attitude really can help.

3. Read books or listen to tapes that focus on coping skills (some are suggested in the Resources section at the back of this book). New ideas ease the tension and fear even if you do not feel they relate directly to your situation.

4. Read the following selections from "Part Two: The Guide" (page 78)—"Visualization," "Challenges/Adventure," "Peace," "Constructive Denial," "The Unknown," "Self-Help," and "Inner Quiet."

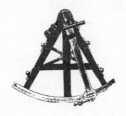

Windless Straits: Boredom and Apathy

You may find yourself becalmed and drifting aimlessly in Windless Straits. The straits symbolize boredom and apathy, in which you have no sense of movement toward any goal. There is a real danger of staying immobilized in these straits unless you generate some activity.

You cannot wait for the winds to come up, for the outside environment to give you direction. You must ignite your own internal engines and initiate the change yourself.

Boredom

Boredom occasionally affects all of us, but when you are physically limited, even temporarily, boredom can become chronic and dangerous. You must take control of your ship's rudder and consult your compass to avoid drifting on the open seas.

Boredom: Warning Signs

1. You find you are watching television more than usual, whether you are interested in it or not.

2. You seem to be staring at—but not seeing—your environment.

3. You rarely initiate any activity.

4. You find reasons to stay in one place, avoiding movement and variety.

5. You keep thinking, "There's nothing to do."

6. You see the future as a big nothing-to-do place.

Boredom: What to Do

1. Become involved in a support group or education program where you can discuss your feelings and learn about your illness.

2. Listen to motivational audio tapes.

3. Focus on a picture—a photograph, a painting—and make up a story. Try it! Get the creative juices flowing. Record it in your Captain's Log (page 128).

4. Keep in touch with things that have always interested you. Keep your mind active. Renew interests and hobbies you were previously too busy to do.

5. Read biographies of people like J. F. Kennedy, Helen Keller, F. D. Roosevelt, and others with impressive accomplishments despite physical problems.

6. Ask for help in getting out of your everyday setting. Go to a park, a shop, or for a drive. Keep yourself open to variety.

7. Read "Part Five: Your Personal Support Group" (page 144) and think about how members cope with their situations.

8. In "Part Two: The Guide" (page 78), read "Boredom," "Goals/Accomplishments," "Self-Help," "The Unknown," "Thinking/Feeling," and "Visualization."

Apathy

When we face an experience that seems totally negative and overwhelming, we may react with apathy. It becomes too complex to sort out our own feelings, much less express our thoughts and feelings to others. Apathy is an easy way out. We disconnect ourselves from our situation and from our normal activities. We "embalm" ourselves. Simon and Garfunkel wrote about this kind of stoicism in their song, "I Am a Rock."

Apathy: Warning Signs

1. You find yourself thinking, "What's the use?"

2. You tell yourself there is nothing you can do about your situation.

3. You tell yourself you no longer care.

4. You want to "just get it over with."

5. Your interest in life has faded.

6. You snarl at others when they attempt to "snap you out of it."

Apathy: What to Do

1. Open yourself to your feelings. You may think you've buried them, but they will resurface at unexpected moments. You will do better to face them while you can build a supportive environment for yourself.

2. Think about those you care for and who care for you. Your closing them out will hurt them even more than losing you.

3. Seek help from a close friend, a member of the clergy, a counselor or other professional.

4. Reward yourself for progress you make toward ridding yourself of apathy. Even if you cry, it's better to experience your situation actively than to avoid it.

5. Make a list of things you gain by being apathetic—for example, not having to talk about your feelings with others, not making decisions, not hurting when sad feelings arise. Seek more positive ways to deal with these same issues. Talk with others who are learning to recognize and accept their feelings. Ask for help in decision-making. Make sure you experience happy and fulfilling feelings as well as sad ones.

6. Seek out others who are in need of help and offer whatever assistance you can. Get ideas from your local chapter of the American Cancer Society (or the support organization for whatever illness you're coping with).

7. Become involved!

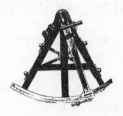

Jagged Rocks: Confusion, Disappointment, and Frustration

The Jagged Rocks are known hazards to beware and steer clear of. These rocks symbolize negative emotions—like confusion, frustration, and disappointment—which snag you, keeping you in one place while the waters swirl around you and move on.

Look into the resources in your ship's hold and find the assertiveness to avoid these Jagged Rocks. Use your telescope to spot the hazards and chart your course away from them.

Confusion

When many powerful events occur in a short period of time, it is common to be confused. But lingering confusion can totally disorient and immobilize you. Your power to make decisions and your sense of control over the events of your life vanish. Be alert to the warning signs and take decisive action to change your course immediately.

Confusion: Warning Signs

1. You seem unable to make decisions about even minor issues in your life.

2. When you finally do make a decision, you continue to worry that it is not the right one.

3. You find you are emotionally paralyzed and unable to sort out how you are feeling.

4. What's most important of all—you're afraid to ask doctors and nurses questions about your cancer or their plans to treat it.

Confusion: What to Do

1. When you visit your physician, have a family member or trusted friend with you to remind you of questions you wish to ask and to corroborate the information you receive.

2. Avoid "my doctor did this" stories, or tales of horror from an acquaintance who happens to know someone with your illness. Without all the facts, secondhand stories just add to the confusion.

3. Ask questions. It's your body. You have a right to know what is going on. But remember, you might not like the answers. Try to be mentally and emotionally prepared for the responses you get. If at all possible, have someone you care about with you.

4. Write down your questions before visiting your doctor, so you won't forget to get the information you need.

5. Don't be embarrassed if you don't understand the first time you're told something about the disease or the

treatment. Ask again. You're not expected to be a medical expert.

6. Don't be afraid of upsetting your physician or nurse by asking questions. Assure them that you're not questioning their ability but are trying to better understand what is happening to you.

7. Don't hesitate to get a second opinion if you think it is necessary. A reputable physician will not be upset by this. But do beware of "shopping around," in order to hear what you want to hear. Check with an oncologist, a cancer specialist.

8. Get as much information on your illness as possible. Check for brochures from the American Cancer Society and the National Cancer Institute. Attend educational programs and tune in to them on television and radio. And remember that you are not an expert. Ask your physician to clarify any points you don't understand.

9. Read and complete the "Treatment" exercises (page 105).

10. Read "Images," "Self," and "The Unknown," in "Part Two: The Guide."

Family Confusion

We, as a society, are inclined to expect the medical profession to be able to cure all ills. So it may be difficult for those of us who have never experienced a chronic illness to realize that physicians may not always have all the answers. They may admit openly that they cannot explain what is happening in the course of your loved one's illness.

If the person with cancer is participating in an investigative study, additional tests may be required. The diagnostic process can be drawn out and involved. Tests may have to be repeated or sent away—even to another state—for analysis. Results may be slow in coming, while you and your loved one are eager for definite plans of action.

You may get different stories from the numerous specialists who may be involved, and each may suggest a different form of treatment. In all, the situation can be frustrating and confusing, and you need to prepare yourself to deal with it.

Family Confusion: Warning Signs

1. You experience feelings of anger and frustration at the physicians who are treating your loved one.

2. Your frustration may lead to frequent outbursts to the nursing staff about the lack of information or explanation of the treatment program.

3. You have a sense of being out of control and overwhelmed by the complexity of the medical program.

4. You fear the treatment program and the tests.

5. You seek out physicians who will tell you and the person with cancer what you both want to hear.

6. You are tempted by "miracle" cures or treatment programs which fail to show scientifically verifiable results.

Family Confusion: What to Do

1. Be an advocate for your loved one. Make certain that her or his needs are being met.

2. Don't let your fear get a grip on your common sense. Investigate all forms of treatment and check them out—with physicians, people who have been through the treatment programs, the American Cancer Society, and the Better Business Bureau.

3. Make sure your loved one is being treated in a cancer center by oncologists, surgeons, and other physicians who treat many cancer patients. Such a center is apt to give the most up-to-date treatment, which may greatly increase the chances for survival.

4. Don't be afraid to ask questions and demand answers. Make certain you know when the doctor in charge will be available to answer your questions. Phone the doctor if you need to. You are paying the physician for a service—and that includes keeping you informed. Be assertive.

5. It's a good idea to write down your questions and concerns before checking with the physician. You may be misinformed or worrying about things that aren't possible.

6. Obtain as much information as you can about the specific type of cancer that has been diagnosed. Attend education programs and watch media presentations about cancer. Tape what you can to share with the person who has cancer.

7. Don't listen to the many stories others will tell you about cancer. Some may be true, but, unless you're a physician yourself, you're not qualified to make medical comparisons.

8. Always think of the person who has cancer as an individual, not as a statistic. Maintaining a positive attitude and following good medical advice can—and has—overcome many a statistic!

Disappointment and Frustration

Most disappointment and frustration evolve from unmet expectations. What you hope for is up to you. But if your emotional state is entirely dependent upon test results and physicians' statements, you probably have forgotten your own internal resources. You must believe in yourself so that, even if things don't go well, you will survive those times with your spirit alive, ready for the next challenge.

Depend on your ship's sturdy construction and flexibility, and make repairs if necessary.

Disappointment and Frustration: Warning Signs

1. You are constantly looking into the future, to the total exclusion of the present.

2. Or, conversely, you completely block out anything to do with the future because you might be disappointed.

3. You keep pretending that "everything will be all right," when inside you feel just the opposite.

4. You avoid positive feelings because you fear being let down.

5. You are setting unrealistic goals and then sinking emotionally because you are unable to meet them.

6. You believe that only a physical change will make you feel better emotionally.

Disappointment and Frustration:
What to Do

1. Choose your goals carefully. Don't sell yourself short, but at the same time don't set goals for yourself that are not possible.

2. Talk to someone you trust about your feelings. Those who are closely involved with you may not be able to separate their own feelings of disappointment and frustration from what you are experiencing. So it's helpful to share how you feel with another who can give you a realistic view. Try discussing your concerns with someone not directly involved in your situation: another person with cancer, a counselor or social worker, a member of the clergy, or—perhaps most helpful of all—someone who has had experience working with people who have cancer.

3. Read "Goals/Accomplishments," "Constructive Denial," "Thinking/Feeling," "The Unknown," "Images," "Self," "Inner Quiet," and "Challenges/Adventure" in "Part Two: The Guide."

4. Read "Part Four: Peace Supplies" (page 132). Listen to audio tapes designed for relaxation and meditation. Focus on letting go of your disappointment and frustration and building new, more realistic expectations.

5. Give yourself credit for all you have managed to do. Be aware of your accomplishments and write them down in your Captain's Log.

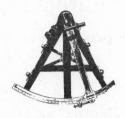

The Void of Silence:
Fear and Despair

The Void of Silence, which encompasses fear and despair, is one of the most difficult and dangerous areas of your journey. Fear and despair are sometimes overwhelming and can swamp you if you are not alert to their warning signs. It will require all your courage and love and belief in yourself to avoid sinking into this void.

Fear

Fear is a normal reaction to cancer, but you cannot allow this feeling to take control of your life. It's natural to fear that which threatens you with pain, loss, and uncertainty about your future. But it's not natural for you to permit this feeling to dominate all other emotions so that pleasure and peace are lost. Move past this fear and continue upon your journey.

Seek out the peaceful inner space of your ship and light the lantern of your inner being for the comfort you need.

Fear: Warning Signs

1. You are continually preoccupied with the future—and you dread it.

2. You interpret everything that happens in a negative way.

3. You speculate on "what ifs" and feel paralyzed—for example, "What if I get my hopes up and things get worse?" or "What if I start doing things for myself and I get hurt?"

4. You lack awareness of anything positive happening to you in the present.

5. You are afraid to believe in anything.

6. You imagine that every little physical sensation is the cancer growing.

7. You find yourself constantly thinking about death but you are afraid to come to grips with it.

Fear: What to Do

1. Focus every day on positive things. View the slightest progress as moving in the right direction. Record it in your Captain's Log.

2. Tell yourself good things. Avoid thoughts like "I'll never get better" or "I'm doomed—why even try?" Instead think, "I feel a little better today," "I sat up for five minutes without getting exhausted," "I walked to the mailbox today—last week I only made it to the kitchen."

3. Talk to someone you feel comfortable with—someone who is supportive and a good listener, but who will not say, "Oh, don't worry, everything will be all right."

4. Investigate your fears. You may be worrying about things that will never happen!

5. Laugh! Find humor or create it. Fear has trouble surviving with humor around.

6. Read and meditate upon the positive thoughts in "Part Four: Peace Supplies."

7. Read the discussion about helplessness and spirituality in "Part Five: Your Personal Support Group."

8. Read "Fear," "The Unknown," "Visualization," "Inner Quiet," "Goals/Accomplishments," "Thinking/Feeling," "Peace," "Prayer," "Life/Death," and "Constructive Denial" in "Part Two: The Guide."

Family Fear

Fear is a powerful emotion. When we are close to a person who has cancer, we are afraid both for the person with cancer and for ourselves. "Will he die?" "Have I done all I can possibly do to ensure the best treatment for her?" "How will I survive without my loved one?" "What do I say to him?" "How do I treat her normally?" If you allow it, your life will be controlled by your fears, and you and the person with cancer both lose. You must take action!

Family Fear: Warning Signs

1. You find you are constantly concerned about the future, usually beginning your thoughts with "what if."

2. You find nothing positive to think about in the present or the future. You cannot shake loose the idea that cancer is always a death sentence.

29

3. You dwell on the possible death of your loved one, even though the person is well and there is no indication that death is imminent or expected.

4. You interpret all the medical information you receive in a negative way, yet never dare ask for specifics to clarify your interpretation.

5. You have lost sight of hope.

Family Fear: What to Do

1. Look for good statistics. If your loved one has a 3 percent chance of cure, you have every right to hope that he or she will be in that category.

2. Recognize progress, no matter how small, and comment on it to others.

3. Make sure any information you receive is accurate and that you check it with the oncologist.

4. Make realistic plans with your loved one. This may include discussions about things the person would like done if he or she dies.

5. Practice a little constructive denial. Read "Constructive Denial" in "Part Two: The Guide."

6. Find other families—in waiting rooms, hospitals, support groups—who are dealing with similar situations. Share your fears and the ways you cope with them. Listen to how others cope and try their methods.

7. Don't eliminate all other aspects of your life. Maintain as much of your normal lifestyle as possible. Quality of time—not quantity—spent with your loved one is most important.

Despair

Despair is not giving up on survival, but rather giving up on yourself. There is a big difference between accepting death, when that is appropriate, and giving up on life. Despair can grow gradually out of depression or descend quickly when you receive bad news. Sometimes despair just appears for no apparent reason. Only an overriding belief in the strength of your spirit—however you define that spirit—and in the ongoing power of loving and caring will help you through this void.

This is more than a life-and-death issue. It concerns the quality of life you choose. Even in the worst of times you have a direct influence on how that life-quality thrives. It is under your control. Focus on your individuality and your inner strength.

Despair: Warning Signs

1. You have little or no interest in what is going on around you.

2. You experience an empty, powerless feeling that persists over long periods of time.

3. You show little or no positive attempts to make contact with other people, even your family.

4. You feel that you are waiting for the worst that can happen to you.

5. You feel drained. You lack energy.

6. If you have counted on your religion, you feel a sense of betrayal, that somehow "God tricked me."

7. Your sense of hope is gone. You feel abandoned.

Despair: What to Do

1. Talk to someone you trust. You may not want to discuss your feelings with anyone, but do it anyway; it's an important step in breaking out of your despair. If despair has been a predominant feeling for you, you would be wise to seek out the help of a professional—a counselor, social worker, or psychologist.

2. Write down the names of people you have touched during your life and can still touch. Record this here or in your Captain's Log. Ask for help from friends and family in this exercise.

3. Accept the love that others are giving you. And let others know you love them.

4. Remember, as long as you are alive you can still make a difference if you choose to. A smile, a touch, a gesture—all are important ways to express caring to others.

5. Write in your Captain's Log daily. Even if you've had a bad day, find at least one positive item to record.

6. Read your Captain's Log and focus on the progress you have made and the help you have received.

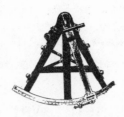

Sandbars of Embarrassment and Guilt

The Sandbars represent some of the more subtle feelings you may experience on your journey—like embarrassment and guilt. These are feelings not usually associated with cancer. And because they are not anticipated, you can be hopelessly stranded on these sandbars before you know it. Whether the sandbars represent a minor annoyance or a major obstacle for you, you must keep a sharp lookout for these avoidable barriers. They can trick you; they lie just below the surface, barely visible until you run aground on them.

The best way to steer clear of the sandbars is to study the charts of those who have traveled this course before you.

Embarrassment

Whenever there is any physical change—seen or unseen—there is the potential for embarrassment. This feeling, often unexpected, can be incapacitating. Embarrassment can limit your interractions with other people at a time when human contact is necessary for your emotional health.

Embarrassment is not caused by the physical changes themselves, but by what you tell yourself about them. If you tell yourself positive things, you will be able to avoid this sandbar. But you must initiate the power to free yourself.

Embarrassment: Warning Signs

1. You are constantly preoccupied with physical changes in yourself.

2. You think self-defeating thoughts like "I look awful!" or "I am no longer a real man (or a real woman)."

3. You continually try to figure out what others are thinking about you—and assume they are thinking the worst.

4. You limit your activities because you feel you will be the object of ridicule, pity, or gossip.

5. You reject all cosmetic solutions because "everyone will know anyway" or "it just isn't the same."

6. You don't want to see visitors, including members of your family.

Embarrassment: What to Do

1. Trust the people who care about you. Your love and inner being are more important to them than how you look.

2. Practice making positive statements to yourself, like, "This wig doesn't look half-bad!" or "I am still the person I have always been inside."

3. See how many people you can brighten up each day with a compliment or a joke.

4. Find photographs or paintings you think are beautiful and reflect on what real beauty is.

5. Get help from others. Find people with a flair for flattering clothing or cosmetics who can advise you on how to enhance your good points to draw attention away from your physical problems. Don't be stopped by the all-too-common attitude that "this is not worth the effort because I have cancer." This is a time when you need as much support and positive activity as possible.

6. Read "Beauty" (page 137) in "Part Four: Peace Supplies."

7. Talk to others who have dealt with some of the physical changes you are experiencing and find out how they helped themselves.

8. Support others who, like you, are struggling with physical problems. You'll be helping yourself as well.

9. Read "Self," "Challenges/Adventure," "Self-Help," "Images," and "Thinking/Feeling" in "Part Two: The Guide" (page 78).

Guilt

It's not unusual for you as a person with cancer to feel guilty that people are "waiting on you"—to believe that you're a burden to others. You may even dredge up a "reason" why you have the disease, based on some presumed wrongdoing in your past. While some of these feelings are natural and represent an attempt to gain some control over your situation, guilt can overwhelm you and disrupt your relationships with your family and your friends.

You may need to make some repairs to your ship, then light your inner lantern and allow it to shine out as a sign of welcome to those near you.

Guilt: Warning Signs

1. You try to do things for yourself that you obviously cannot do, risking injury to yourself.

2. To avoid being a burden, you do not tell people of your needs and therefore deprive them of opportunities to help you.

3. You invent reasons to keep visitors away so they won't be saddened at how you have changed.

4. You are preoccupied with how difficult it is for your spouse or parent or anyone who is caring for or assisting you. Instead of focusing on getting well, you mull over what a chore caring for you must be.

5. You refuse to accept the idea that those who love you get pleasure from caring for you.

6. You scan the events of your past, dwelling on your mistakes and mentally punishing yourself as if your cancer were retribution for those mistakes.

Guilt: What to Do

1. Remember that if you feel you are not giving enough, you can focus on giving your love. It is the best gift of all.

2. Remind yourself that when you helped others you did it because you cared for them. You did not think of them as "burdens."

3. Be creative. Think of ways you can help others each day.

4. Talk over your feelings with people with whom you feel comfortable. Gain their perspective on the situation. Ask for ways you can contribute so that you feel less helpless.

5. Think of all the things you have done to help others and focus on your positive accomplishments. You may need some help rounding out this positive picture of yourself—from family, friends, counselors, clergy.

6. Read "Part Five: Your Personal Support Group" and learn how others deal with guilt. Also read "Communication" and "Helplessness" (pages 157 and 149) in Part Five.

7. Read "Part Four: Peace Supplies" and meditate on more positive and helpful thoughts. You have today to begin anew.

8. In "Part Two: The Guide," work on the Thinking/Feeling Exercises. Read "Self," "Goals/Accomplishments," "Self-help," "Inner Quiet."

Family Guilt

Guilt often accompanies other feelings. For instance, you may feel guilty that you are sometimes angry with the person who has cancer for not contributing as much as he or she once did to the household, child care, or finances. If the person's cancer is advanced, you feel guilty for thinking that death might be a release from suffering. Conversely, your desire for the person with cancer to go on living, even while suffering, produces guilt feelings too.

Perhaps it's necessary for you to become involved in financial issues related to the person's death—and you feel guilty for bringing up the subject of money as if you were doing it out of greed.

If you don't counteract your feelings of guilt, they will permeate your extire existence for the duration of the cancer and beyond. You may live with this feeling for the rest of your life. Guilt accomplishes nothing—except to keep you zeroed in on yourself and alienated from the person you care about.

Family Guilt: Warning Signs

1. You feel frustrated because you can't do enough or aren't strong enough to cope with the situation.

2. You don't talk about your daily activities or about having a pleasant time because your family member is homebound and not feeling well.

3. You feel guilty for wanting some time alone.

4. You feel guilty simply because you are well. You don't want to eat or are unable to sleep because your loved one is having difficulty eating or sleeping.

Family Guilt: What to Do

1. Take the "shoulds" and "shouldn'ts" out of your thinking: "I should be able to...," "I shouldn't feel this way," or "I shouldn't have said that."

2. Be more aware of what is important in your relationship—of what you are doing that is valuable.

3. Don't accept the idea that you cannot help the way you feel. You are in control of your thoughts. Pay attention to what you are thinking, and you can help pull yourself off this sandbar. Read "Thinking/Feeling" in "Part Two: The Guide."

4. Remember that the person who has cancer often feels guilty too. Have open discussions with this person about the guilt you are feeling. If this is difficult for you, ask for help from a counselor, a member of the clergy, or your support group.

5. Notice all the positive things you do for others. Give yourself a little reward for doing these things. Focus on what you can do, and let what you can't do slide from your awareness.

6. Listen to audio tapes on relaxation to help you ease up and think positive thoughts.

7. If you believe you are not doing enough, ask for feedback from others. If you truly cannot accomplish all that needs doing, ask for help. Be specific as to what you need done, when, and how often.

8. Read about guilt and communication in "Part Five: Your Personal Support Group."

9. Read "Family/Friends Exercise," "Goals/Accomplishments," and "Self-Help" in "Part Two: The Guide."

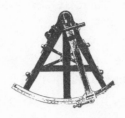

The Speechless Triangle: Overprotection

This part of the journey is where family communication systems—the ways family members usually talk to each other about important subjects—often break down. One cause is overprotection—reluctance to talk about the cancer and its effects with the person who has it and others closely involved.

Even in families that ordinarily have good communication systems, the great strain of dealing with cancer can cause communications to become fragmented and scattered. Your relationships may be in peril. At the very least, you are unable to enjoy the open sharing you once did. When family members stop sharing with each other, mutual understanding can become almost impossible. It's up to you to let your love and caring overcome the resistance to communicate honestly. Talking about cancer is always difficult, but it can be done.

Overprotection

People who care about each other naturally want to protect each other, but this strategy of protection, when used excessively, tends to stifle communication and sharing.

Trust that those you care about can handle the bad times. And face these bad times together, as a team. Be as open and honest with each other as you have been through other difficult situations. The strength of your relationship has come from that openness and honesty.

Fly your ship's flags high; let your signals be clear.

Overprotection: Warning Signs

1. You hold back more and more information about your condition, needs, and emotions from those closest to you.

2. You do not share your feelings with them.

3. You want to talk openly about your feelings and your relationships, but you just don't get around to it. Instead, you talk about the weather or any other "safe" topic.

4. You constantly worry about saying the "wrong thing."

5. You feel "phony" about the time you spend with the people who love you, and you begin to dread that time because of the charade involved.

6. You have needs that a concerned person could meet, but you don't ask because she or he "has enough to worry about."

Overprotection: What to Do

1. Since you're not communicating effectively, find an intermediary to help you (counselor, clergyperson, support group).

2. Trust each other to handle whatever comes along. Don't interpret another person's feelings before you know what they really are.

3. Visualize yourself together on this sea journey, working as a close-knit crew, a source of strength for each other.

4. Touch each other. It is a powerful form of communication.

5. If you can, take courses and read books on improving communication skills. Effective communication may sound simple, but it takes thought and practice. (See the "Resources" on pages 183-185 or ask your librarian or bookseller for help.)

6. In "Part Five: Your Personal Support Group," read what others in your situation have said about communication.

7. Read "Thinking/Feeling," "Fear," and "Self" in "Part Two: The Guide."

Family Overprotection

The diagnosis of cancer can make normal communications between family members stiff and lacking in genuine sharing. Family members wonder if the person with cancer should be told about his or her illness, how much to tell the children, what distant relatives and friends should know. They wonder if they themselves—the close family members—even have the full story. Family members may receive differing bits of information from physicians. Communication—or lack of it—may turn into a game. And soon the entire family may be caught up in subterfuge that could put any spy mystery to shame!

Family Overprotection: Warning Signs

1. You aren't sure who knows what and how much. Therefore you avoid talking to certain members of the family. When you talk, you feel they can see the lie in your eyes.

2. You have an uncomfortable feeling about how little some members of the family know about the illness. You wonder what their reaction might be if something serious should happen.

3. You begin to structure elaborate visitation schedules and rules to limit the amount of time certain persons spend with your loved one. These rules are not related to the physical condition or the requests of the person with cancer. Instead, they reflect your own wish to protect him or her.

4. You are unable to talk openly to the person with cancer. Since you feel uncomfortable with the subject of cancer, you avoid it at all costs, even switching off the television if the word is mentioned. You may even ask medical personnel not to mention the word.

5. You think about the possibility of the person's dying. You have many feelings you want to express, and yet you can't discuss this possibility. You fear that just talking about it will imply that you have given up, which will be upsetting or depressing to the person with cancer.

Family Overprotection: What to Do

1. Drop the charade! It won't work, and it's a handicap! You'll probably need outside help to accomplish this, so ask for it—from a trusted friend, a priest, minister, or rabbi, a social worker, nurse, or physician.

2. Be kind to yourself; understand that the stress of your situation has led to your overprotective attitudes and actions. But be firm in eliminating them.

3. Realize that what you are doing is really not protecting the person with cancer. People have an innate sense of physical self and usually are aware of their own states of health—sometimes even before the diagnoses are made. Keeping secrets or avoiding the subject is just silencing any form of communication you may be able to have.

4. Be open with children. They are experts at reading nonverbal communication and are aware of much more than you imagine. Also, they often worry more about the situation than you realize. If you don't allow them to ask questions and get true answers, they may develop unfounded fears and become more upset than if you were honest with them from the start. If you are open with them, you provide them with an opportunity to discuss their feelings with you. You may need help with this; ask someone you trust.

5. If children or other adults ask if the person with cancer is going to die, you can respond with: "It is a possibility, but there are other possibilities too." Then look at how the child or adult is handling the situation now; focus on the present, not the future.

6. Understand that being honest does not mean being blunt or tactless or unkind. It means discussing real events and projected events and sharing emotional reactions to those events.

7. Start slowly. Discussions about truly important issues—no matter what they may be—are always difficult. So don't rush. And don't let silences scare you away from the

issues. It's often hard to find the right words to describe feelings. Be persistent.

8. Listen. Don't interpret another's response and then change it into something it wasn't meant to be. If you're uncertain about the meaning of what's said to you, just ask for clarification.

9. Be honest. Don't pretend that you're not concerned or afraid—or angry, if you are. Try to explain what you are really feeling to the person with cancer or another family member. Allow that person to help you.

10. Talking about death can be hard for everyone. The point is to talk about your feelings. "I am afraid of losing you" is a way to express your concern that your loved one may die. The important thing is to let your loved one know how much you care.

11. If it seems useful, seek help from a nonfamily member to guide the conversation.

12. If you need to make financial arrangements, do it together, as it involves both of you: "If something happens to either of us, we need to get this taken care of."

13. Read "Family/Friends Exercise" and "Constructive Denial" in "Part Two: The Guide."

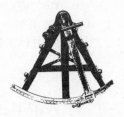

Rapids of Helplessness

The Rapids of Helplessness are a special challenge on your journey. When you're running these rapids, you feel that you're being rushed along at a breakneck pace and that, no matter how hard you struggle, there is no escape. You are not in control. You are in a nightmare, yet you're awake. This is frightening.

Only a powerful belief in yourself and your spirit—in your ship and your buoyancy—can get you through. But you can do it! The rapids will end. You can learn how to survive until calmer waters appear.

Helplessness

Helplessness is a natural reaction to the news that you have cancer. Your body seems to be betraying you by not doing what you want it to do. Nurses and doctors are examining you, giving you orders, and moving you around from test to test. Family members are taking over tasks and responsibilities that you feel you should be doing. It's easy to feel that you are no longer in control of your life.

47

Now is the time to realize that you are only as helpless as you believe you are. You must have confidence that you are built of strong and flexible stuff that can withstand the rigors of the rapids.

Helplessness: Warning Signs

1. You find you are constantly thinking about what you can't do.

2. You have strong feelings of frustration slowly changing to apathy.

3. You say, "There's nothing I can do" or "It's in the doctor's hands now" or "It's God's will."

4. Your moods swing between panic and depression. You feel totally defeated.

5. You no longer question what is being done for you or to you by the medical staff.

6. You let others do things for you that you could do for yourself if you tried.

7. Or—just the opposite—you're constantly proving you're not helpless by doing things you cannot safely do.

8. You have lost sight of your personal power. You feel you are being endlessly drawn toward total defeat.

Helplessness: What to Do

1. Focus on the things you *are* able to do. Make a list of these things and add to it. Ask for ideas on how others see you.

2. Allow others to help you when you need it. Remember that by allowing them to help you, you are really helping them to feel useful.

3. Remind yourself that helplessness is a state of mind, not of body. There are many people with extensive physical limitations who do not consider themselves helpless and who make major contributions to their families and to society.

4. Try to avoid contact with people who promote your helplessness, no matter how well-meaning they may be. They may do "everything" for you, or treat you like a spoiled child, saying yes to your every whim because you are ill. They may treat you like a victim, not encouraging you to do better, assuming you are going to fail. You don't need this kind of relationship. You need all the encouragement and support you can get!

5. Seek out sources of courage and strength for yourself. It may be a friend who has had experiences that parallel yours, a book about someone who overcame great odds with courage, a seminar or group, or any other personal resource you may have.

6. Use humor to help you. Find things to laugh at. This includes yourself, now and then, if you need to poke holes in your constant seriousness.

7. Give yourself credit for the attempts you make to cope or to improve, even if they're not always successful.

8. Read "Thinking/Feeling," "Challenges/Adventure," "Constructive Denial," "Inner Quiet," "The Unknown," "Prayer," "Life/Death," and "Goals/Accomplishments" in "Part Two: The Guide."

9. Read "Part Five: Your Personal Support Group" and pay attention to how members deal with feelings of helplessness.

Helplessness: Family

One of the most difficult things for anyone is to watch someone they love become disabled by illness. It can become extremely frustrating to be unable to contribute anything tangible to that person's healing. The more serious the illness and the less favorable the prognosis, the harder it is to find ways to help. Helplessness is a natural reaction to such circumstances. That feeling can be so overpowering that merely visiting the person becomes an uncomfortable task. For close family members, helplessness can lead to bitterness, anger, depression, and even physical illness.

It is most important to examine your feelings and your capabilities, and then to set realistic goals for yourself. If you concentrate on what you *can* do—not on what you can't—you will ride out these rapids.

Family Helplessness: Warning Signs

1. You feel you are "banging your head against a stone wall," as if all your efforts are futile.

2. This feeling of futility can lead to apathy: "It's no use. I just don't care anymore."

3. You are "running yourself into the ground," doing all your usual tasks in addition to caring for the person with cancer and handling the duties that person normally performed.

4. You have thoughts of leaving the situation—just walking away. Then you're remorseful about even thinking such a thing.

5. You find yourself frantically anticipating all possible situations and devising strategies to deal with each one.

6. If you try to pull away from this accelerated pace, the feeling of helplessness intensifies.

Family Helplessness: What to Do

1. Change your focus from what you are not able to do to what you can accomplish. And don't expect yourself to accomplish things with the same quality and attention to detail as you would normally.

2. It's critical that you understand that you are making a difference, that the situation is better because you are involved. Don't downplay your contributions because they seem to be less than you wish they were, or because the cancer is not "cured." Don't minimize the importance of caring relationships and the power of love.

3. Measure your importance to the other person in terms of that person's quality of life. You cannot directly influence the amount of time the person will survive.

4. Open yourself to suggestions from others—including the person who has cancer—on how you can contribute.

5. Look for opportunities to renew yourself. See a movie or a play or take part in other activities that are rewarding to you.

6. Accept praise and compliments on the things that you accomplish.

7. Involve the person with cancer in any tasks in which he or she can participate. By sharing in activities, you both will feel a sense of accomplishment and control.

8. Keep yourself medically informed. Know about the type of cancer your loved one has and its treatment. Ask

questions and act as an advocate. Be present, if you can, when the person meets with physicians and other treatment providers.

9. In "Part Two: The Guide," read "Family/Friends Exercise," "Goals/Accomplishments," "Images," and "Inner Quiet."

10. Read in "Part Five: Your Personal Support Group" about helplessness (page 149).

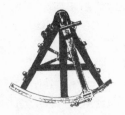

Whirlpools of Anger and Depression

Whirlpools are emotional maelstroms. They represent feelings of anger and depression, which pull you down deeper and deeper at an ever-increasing speed. When you are facing cancer, you are pulled into whirlpools almost before you know it, and you find yourself in a downward spiral. These emotions of anger and depression, which seem to dominate all others, can consume you. The deeper you are in the whirlpool, the harder it is to break out and resurface.

It's better to be aware of these whirlpools than to try to ignore them. Though you probably can't avoid them completely, you can skirt their edges and not get sucked into their powerful downcurrents.

Anger

You have many things to feel angry about. You must do things you don't want to do. You must tell people unpleasant news. You must endure pain and discomfort with no guarantee of a cure. Anger is a common response for people who have cancer, but anger is not something you can hold on to for long. It can pull you down and keep you there. When you need your energy to fight for your life, you may be dissipating it by being angry.

You must catch the winds of motivation and hold your rudder steady to pull yourself from this whirlpool.

Anger: Warning Signs

1. You feel constantly angry—a slow, internal simmer.

2. You relive long-past situations that made you angry, and revive those past feelings of anger.

3. Frequently you find yourself verbally attacking people you care about over issues that are insignificant.

4. You block out positive feelings. You rarely laugh or smile. In fact, you prefer to scowl.

5. Your anger is turning into bitterness, a penetrating feeling that chills your entire life.

6. You actively fight feelings of joy, avoiding occasions that could bring you joy.

7. You are holding the anger inside you, even though you may appear calm on the outside.

8. You snap at people in general, from store clerks to the nurses in your clinic.

Anger: What to Do

1. Talk about your feelings with someone you trust. Choose someone you can feel comfortable with while

expressing your angry feelings. Make sure that this person will keep your conversation confidential. You may want to consult a professional counselor or a support group.

2. Ask yourself if being angry is helping you. If not, replace it with a more positive feeling, like love. Of course, it is difficult to do, but you are fighting for your life and your quality of life.

3. Listen to audio tapes that can bring you peacefulness and relaxation.

4. Use your anger as energy to spur you into activity. Research your situation. Volunteer to help others. Exercise. Knit. Construct. Paint. Do anything that will rechannel your thoughts into something constructive.

5. Read "Part Five: Your Personal Support Group" and listen to how group members handled their anger.

6. In "Part Two: The Guide," read "Thinking/Feeling," "Peace," and "Inner Quiet."

Anger: Family

The experience of cancer is frustrating, and anger is a common reaction. Anger is a particularly confusing emotion for family members, who don't believe they are "allowed" to be angry at the person with cancer. If they do get angry, they feel guilty about it. Therefore, family members often suppress their angry feelings. For instance, a husband may be angry because his wife is sick and can't perform the tasks that contribute to the family's smooth functioning. And yet his anger makes no sense to him because, after all, his wife did not get cancer on purpose. Usually, family members don't admit this anger to themselves or anybody else, just because it sounds selfish. Sometimes they will go to the extreme of never showing anger to the person with cancer, even when the person's behavior becomes childish or obnoxious. Suppressing anger may work for a while, but as the anger builds, it may resurface at unexpected times and in uncontrolled ways. Sometimes anger can be directed at the cancer itself, at the medical profession, or at some person who causes the uneasiness of family members.

It's important to examine your angry feelings honestly, realize the source of your anger, then try to express your anger in constructive ways.

Family Anger: Warning Signs

1. You find yourself continually accepting behavior in the person who has cancer that you wouldn't have tolerated when he or she was well. You excuse the behavior with, "Oh, well, it's just the cancer."

2. Your relationship with this person is strained. You feel you have a pasted-on smile most of the time.

3. Your temper is short; you snap at anyone or anything around you. When you vent your anger, it's in an inappropriate tirade.

4. You feel alone, that you're the only person in the world with such a burden to contend with.

5. You feel you must always be available to others, with little or no time to yourself. And you resent it!

6. You constantly feel as though you want to escape your

situation. You plan ways to leave or to rid yourself of your overwhelming responsibilities.

7. You get furious at others who "have it easy."

8. You feel you must always be in control of your emotions, always present the "proper" image.

9. You find it impossible to enjoy anything.

Family Anger: What to Do

1. First, admit your anger. Realize that there is nothing "wrong" or "stupid" about feeling angry. Many people are angry when faced with similar circumstances. Accept your anger, and then want to let go of it.

2. Talk about your feelings with a "neutral" person who will listen and give you an honest response. Sometimes the real source of our anger is clouded, and other times we have a clear right to be angry. It's hard to sort out these issues without help.

3. Remember, once you admit to yourself that you are angry, you have the responsibility of letting it go. When you're unaware of your anger or disguise it from yourself, you cling to it.

4. Anger can be entangled with self-righteousness, and this combination can make ridding yourself of anger nearly impossible. Accept fault in others and learn to forgive. Even the most justified anger doesn't help anyone. Look at your situation objectively, and then try to find constructive ways to alter it.

5. If your angry feelings run deep, you may need professional help in coping with them. Don't be afraid to ask for it.

6. Listen to audio tapes that emphasize meditation and relaxation. Focus on maintaining a feeling of peace even while thinking of those things you became angry about in the past.

7. Read "Part Five: Your Personal Support Group" and find out how others deal with anger.

8. In "Part Two: The Guide," read "Thinking/Feeling," "Challenges/Adventure," and "The Unknown."

Depression

Feeling sad or down from time to time is normal for all of us. When the diagnosis is cancer, a common reaction is sadness and a sense of loss. But being depressed is different from just being sad. Depression permeates your whole existence and causes a devastating emotional paralysis which can sink you if you're not prepared.

You need to set your sails to catch the breezes of motivation and activate your internal energy source to pull yourself out of this dangerous whirlpool.

Depression: Warning Signs

1. You lack motivation to do even simple tasks.

2. You have frequent crying spells over an extended period of time.

3. You feel that you are abandoned by family, friends, physicians.

4. You let yourself neglect personal hygiene—bathing, shaving, nail care. Many mornings you choose not to get dressed.

5. You experience wide mood swings, from total despair to euphoric confidence.

6. You block out positive feelings. You convince yourself that your situation is so bleak that you can't feel good ever again.

7. You find yourself thinking, maybe even saying, "What's the use?"

8. Since you feel that your future can never improve and will only get worse, you constantly dwell on the past.

Depression: What to Do

1. Don't keep thinking about what you've lost. Think of what you still have and what you have gained by your experiences. You may find you have a great deal to offer others.

2. Keep your mind active. Go to movies. Read. Listen to music. Enjoy the company of interesting, stimulating people. Try to spend less time dwelling on your own situation.

3. Listen to audio tapes that concentrate on positive images. Even if you're not sure they will help—or that you can get well—listen anyway. At least you'll be spending your time in a positive environment.

4. Read "Part Four: Peace Supplies." Find words that can contribute to your sense of peace and well-being.

5. Read "Part Five: Your Personal Support Group" and listen carefully to how members coped with their own depression.

6. In "Part Two: The Guide," read "Inner Quiet," "Images," "Thinking/Feeling," "Visualization," "Challenges/Adventure," and "Goals/Accomplishments."

7. Use the Thinking/Feeling Exercises (page 101) to explore your emotions. It's much easier to solve problems when you know what the problems are.

8. Don't expect too much of yourself. Reward yourself for positive thoughts and activities. But don't be hard on yourself if you do give in to depression now and then. Just gently and persistently draw yourself away from it.

9. Ask for professional help and guidance if you need it to do this successfully.

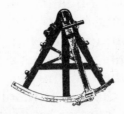

Spirit Islands in the Lake of Strength

In the midst of all the potential traps that await you on your journey, there is a place of hope and sustenance. It is the Lake of Strength. Here, in this spring-fed lake, you begin to find your own peace and courage. Here you feel yourself come alive. You are renewed. You recognize that inside you is the strength you need to complete your journey and reach the Sea of Serenity.

In the Lake of Strength are six small islands, each offering something you need for your journey. You may visit these islands as often as you wish or need to. They are a place within you—a source for the feelings the islands describe. Remember to seek them out when your burden becomes too heavy.

Island of Courage

Probably you have never needed this type of courage before. It's not just the courage to fight *against* someone or something; it's the courage to fight *for* someone and something—yourself and a quality life. It's the courage that comes from trusting yourself, no matter what is happening. To have this kind of courage, you must love yourself and treat yourself with dignity. It takes a special courage to embark on a journey when the means are more important than the end. How the disease is resolved physically—whether by cure or by death—does not make the journey successful or unsuccessful. Rather it's the day-to-day choices, each choice requiring an act of courage, that determine the journey's quality.

The Island of Courage is there. Of that there is no doubt. Your challenge is to discover that courage. The other islands in this Lake of Strength are marked with lighthouses that can guide you in your quest.

Courage: What to Do

1. Go for a walk. Find a smooth rock. Look at it carefully and form an image of it in your mind. This smooth stone feels nice to your fingers. It's cool and hard. It's strong. No matter how hard you press on it, it does not give way. Even something many times its size—like a tree—can fall on it and it will not crack or give way.

Picture your inner strength as this small, smooth stone. No matter what burdens you carry, your strength does not give way. You can seek out your secret strength whenever you need it. Carry your stone with you when you face a situation that demands your strength.

Or substitute another object for the stone. Rosary beads, worry beads, a special ring, or another object may represent your inner strength. Just remember to sense the strength of the object and relate it to your own.

2. Read stories about people who have been courageous in adversity. Picture yourself among those courageous people, possessing the same characteristics, the same inner strength. If you can't get out of the house or the hospital to pick up these biographies, ask others to get the books for you. If reading is hard for you, obtain audio tapes from the library or ask someone to read to you.

3. Seek out others who support you and encourage you to be courageous. Avoid or confront those who treat you as an object of pity. That is a reflection of their own fears and does not help you at all. You may find yourself trying to ease *their* concerns.

This doesn't mean that you should avoid discussing fear and death with those you trust and feel comfortable with. The most courageous person is fearful at times. But talk about these issues from a position of power, like the captain of a ship. Be prepared to make the sacrifices and survive the storm.

4. Don't be afraid to ask for help. We all credit ourselves with being independent. And we would not hesitate to help a friend in need. But when it comes time for us to ask for help and to allow others to help us, we feel guilty about it. In times of crisis, people must depend upon each other.

5. In "Part Two: The Guide," read "Constructive Denial." Picture yourself in a situation in which you will survive by your courage, persistence, and wits. Focus on your situation and see it as a challenge.

Island of Openness

The Island of Openness is a requisite for your journey. You need to be open to explore new alternatives in a variety of areas: personal, business, medical, emotional, financial. This does not mean you have to change your whole life, but rather to be open to change when it presents itself. Viewing new ideas with scorn deprives you of different and perhaps more creative approaches to your problems. Your life is not the same as it used to be. And since your life has changed, your approach to solving the problems of your new life must change as well.

Openness: What to Do

1. Open yourself to new ideas—your own and other people's. Don't close the doors of possibility!

2. Recognize that openness may be painful. Most processes of change and growth involve some pain.

3. Stay flexible. Be open to changing old patterns.

4. Be open to accepting physical help, as well as the love and caring of others.

5. Be open to help wherever you may find it. Help may come from surprising sources.

6. Seek others who are willing to encourage your openness. You'll find many who can't seem to look into your eyes, can't bear to listen to you speak openly about your experiences. Instead, you need those who can sit with you and listen to you. This is a time when only those friends who can offer themselves without reservation will be of real help to you.

7. Be open with yourself. Don't shut out your feelings. Open yourself to your experiences and remain in touch with your options. We feel most lost when we decide we have no options.

8. Share your openness and honesty with those you love and those you encounter, including children and older adults, who are often neglected in the "opening up" process. You can't be the judge of how they will react to the situation. Just as you survived hearing that you had cancer, when you thought you never could, they will undoubtedly be able to handle the honest information you give them. Children are able to respond in a mature and understanding way, and they can comfort you. Older adults are able to share their memories of times when they found inner strength to endure their own trials. There are very few instances in which children and older adults should not be told the facts.

Playing games for the sake of protecting certain persons can be complicated and draining: "You can tell Aunt Anne, but don't tell Bob—he can't take it." "Mom is too frail—we'll have to gloss over the situation for her." "How can I remember who knows what?"

Realize that if people can't handle the truth, they will find their own ways to avoid the situation.

9. If how to tell what to whom becomes a real dilemma for you, ask someone you trust for some advice.

Island of Hope

Hope is often a misunderstood concept when related to the cancer experience. Initially you might think of hope as the desire to get well. But hope is much more than desire; it can't be limited to just "getting what I want." Hope must encompass the effort—including hard work and determination—to reach that goal of wellness. You must be willing to get involved in the process of getting well—by helping yourself physically, emotionally, and spiritually. Hope involves seeing your body, mind, and spirit as a whole being—and your life as an ongoing evolution of growth and increased awareness. Hope looks to the future but rests in the present. It guides your present experience and reflects your love for life.

No matter where you are on your journey, your Island of Hope is your spiritual home, a place in your heart that you never leave for long.

Hope: What to Do

1. Don't let your fears and concerns override your sense of hope. There is nothing wrong with being hopeful; the idea of "false hope" is absurd. Be realistic; be prepared for the worst. But always hope for the best. Like a sea captain facing a hurricane, you recognize the risks and evaluate your chances, but you prepare your vessel and you fight to survive!

2. Use all of your being to fight for getting well. Treating your physical body alone is not enough if your emotional and spiritual selves have "given up." Rest and feed your body well. Get enough exercise. Rest and feed your emotional self and your spiritual self too. Read peaceful, stimulating, hopeful material. Relax and meditate. Visualize yourself getting well and doing all the things you've always wanted to do. If you're telling yourself, "I've *never* been able to do those things—why aim for them now?" begin to realize that you are fighting for your life!

3. Listen to your inner dialogue. What are you focusing on? Steer your thoughts away from all that may be going wrong, your "what ifs," your fears, your dread for the future. Focus on what is going right this very moment. Recognize that you are in control of your thoughts, and use your control to your advantage. Jot down your thoughts in your Captain's Log and work through them, sorting out the negative and keeping the positive.

4. Remember that everyone grounds his or her existence upon hope. No one has any assurance of the length of life. As long as we are alive, we need to acknowledge hope and plan for the future. We hope for the best, setting a course that always includes an Island of Hope.

Island of Love

As surprising as it may seem, the Island of Love is often overlooked as part of the journey—perhaps the most important part! Most people are grateful for love and support from family and friends, but they forget love's depth and power. Love is healing. It helps put together the pieces of a shattered life. The person who has cancer not only needs to receive love, but to give love too. Everyone needs to love others. When you are actively involved in loving, you are involved in your life, and that is healthy. Loving is living.

Love: What to Do

1. Think of all those you love and have loved. Dwell on these caring relationships. Write about them in your Captain's Log.

2. Tell those you love that you love them. Say the words!

3. Picture love as a cloud, a pink, warm cloud that engulfs you, easing pain, fear, and discomfort. This love emanates from God, from your friends, from your family. This love cloud contains all of their caring and hope for your recovery. The cloud fills your personal space. It mists over and hides all other emotions and cares. You are lifted gently above your tired body, and you are able to rest.

4. Practice love. Ask for touches, backrubs, hugs. Do something nice for someone else. Write a poem. Send flowers. Make a card. Read a story aloud.

5. Be aware of loving gestures from those around you. Accept them without guilt or other negative feelings.

6. Read about love and loving relationships, in poetry and prose.

7. Recognize that love can displace fear.

Island of Laughter

This island is a place where laughter reigns. It is a space free of pain and hurt and open to the beauty and simplicity of life. It is a place where there are no restrictions about how to behave—no rules like "Act your age!" or "Be an adult!"

One dictionary defines laughter as a "movement of the muscles of the face, especially the lips, accompanied by an escape of noise from the throat." How inadequate! Laughter is a wonderful musical sound unique to humans. It's an expression of joy and delight, often over life's simple pleasures—good tidings, a child's playtime imagination, or just plain human silliness. Laughter is a salute to the joy of being alive.

Norman Cousins in his book *Anatomy of an Illness* describes how he purposefully induced laughter in himself during a life-threatening illness. He watched "Candid Camera" and other funny television shows and found that for each ten minutes of a good belly laugh he was rewarded with two hours of pain-free relaxation.

Let laughter back into your life! Find that carefree island and visit it when you can. Sure, you are in a "serious situation" and you must "tough it out," but ease that situation by appreciating life's delights and good humor. Celebrate, with laughter, your joy in just being alive.

Laughter: What to Do

1. Plant the garden on your Island of Laughter with the kind of humor that you, personally, prefer. Then cultivate laughter like a prize rose. Spray away the pests of pain and worry. Appreciate your inner joy as it blossoms and grows.

2. Find videos that make you laugh, and watch them regularly.

3. Smile.

4. Read bits of humor—essays, jokes, descriptions—that make you laugh.

5. Write down your own ideas. What is funny to you? Recall some of the funny situations from your own life.

6. Share humor and laughter with those around you.

7. Family members: don't be afraid to laugh. You're allowed to share joy, even in difficult times.

Island of Wellness

When you have cancer and you don't feel well, your thoughts are likely to be centered on your sickness. But you must remember that there is still wellness in your body, and that wellness can be tapped. Focus on that wellness and see it replacing the sickness. Let your wellness be the keel for your spirit. Don't just think about *becoming well*; focus on the wellness that *already exists* within your body. The power of mind and spirit and the will to live are just beginning to be understood, but there is no doubt that they have a tremendous influence on a person's well-being. Learn to take control of that power, and learn to use it to your advantage. Instead of just fighting sickness, you can promote wellness. All your acts should be pointed toward maximizing the wellness within you.

Wellness: What to Do

1. Decide what you mean by wellness. In your Captain's Log, describe yourself as a well person—what you are doing, how you look.

2. Picture yourself as being well. Do not let your illness control your life. If at all possible, continue doing the things you have always done or begin things you have always wanted to do.

3. If you're unable physically to do some things you enjoy doing, picture yourself doing them. For instance, if you like to play golf, picture your favorite golf course, the people you're likely to play with or see. Visualize the kind of day it is. Hear the sounds. Smell the fresh-mown fairways. Feel

your body respond as you play the game. Make your images as real as possible! Really get into it!

4. Exercise your body within the limits of your doctor's advice. Even if you're only doing breathing exercises, or just moving your arms and legs in bed, this can seem as rewarding as a good long hike or run.

5. Eat well. Choose nutritious foods. Enjoy what you eat, and try to make mealtime special or festive. Add a flower or a candle to your table.

6. Laugh as much as possible. Look for humor or create your own.

7. Keep your mind active. Challenge yourself.

8. See your physical, emotional, and spiritual selves working together to make up a whole, well person.

9. Close your eyes and picture a cave on your Island of Wellness. You have never explored it before. See and feel yourself entering the cave and following a clear, easy pathway that descends. You use a strong flashlight to illuminate beautiful cave drawings on the rock walls. A sweet, cool fragrance drifts into your awareness and you see light ahead of you. You switch off your flashlight and continue to descend toward the light, feeling better with each step. Your body feels light and springy. Your breath comes easily. Your skin tingles and is warm.

You enter the bright hole that is the source of the light and fragrance, and you discover yourself in a deep cavern bathed in sunlight coming through the rocky opening above. The sunlight falls on a pond surrounded by the most beautiful flowers you have ever seen. Their fragrance is amazing. The pond is clear and just the right temperature.

You take off your clothes and submerge yourself in this pond of wellness. You may stay there for as long as you like. And you may return to this pond on your Island of Wellness whenever you need to.

10. Seek out accounts of people who have overcome illness and gained wellness. Visualize yourself doing this. Believe in yourself!

Island of Magic

The most mystical of all the islands and certainly the least understood is the Island of Magic. This magic does not involve sleight of hand or tricks with mirrors. Rather it is a *sense of magic*, a belief in the unknown, an appreciation of the awesome power of life and the mystery that surrounds it. The Island of Magic gives rise to children's curiosity and a freshness of spirit that's often lost to cynicism as we grow older. Magic comes from the idea that we are all bound together, sharing joy and pain. If we choose to see our togetherness, we will know that we are not alone. Our belief in a Higher Power, whether we call it God or Life or Oneness, grows on this island. This magic gives us faith in life, in ourselves, and in the unknown.

Magic: What to Do

1. Be playful. Let the child within you out!

2. See the unknown with curiosity rather than fear.

3. Accept the powers that are greater than yourself.

4. Be humble in the knowledge of just how much you do not know.

5. Be excited about how much you can learn—even from having cancer.

6. Pray or meditate or just open yourself to the mystery that is life.

7. Look at the magic of your everyday world: sunrises, flowers, rain, animals, children.

8. Savor life. Bask in its beauty and its magic.

9. Share the magic that is you with those around you.

10. Read sources of inspiration from the East and from the West, like the Bible and the Tao Te Ching.

11. Read books that create an atmosphere of magic for the reader. For example, books by Carlos Castaneda or Jane Roberts' Seth books make for fascinating reading.

12. Pay attention to the symbolism in rituals, holidays, and church or synagogue services which reflect our need to explore the unknown—and to find strength in the magic of our discoveries.

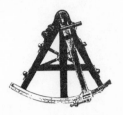

The Sea of Serenity

You have reached your goal, your journey's end. You have overcome the hazards and basked in the joys of your voyage. Now you look back with awe at your accomplishments and how far you have come. You look ahead to the Sea of Serenity, a place where peace reigns. Here, no matter what situation may arise, acceptance and peace prevail.

This is no fairyland, where death and suffering do not exist, but a place where, no matter what the external world's realities may be, the internal world maintains its equilibrium. You can move easily to this place of calm within yourself and remain there for as long as you wish. You have a deep inner confidence that comes from the knowledge that you can endure great hazards and still know what is really important.

Your stay in the Sea of Serenity holds no promises that you will remain there forever. You may find that you drift back into rougher seas from time to time. But each time it is easier to return to this peaceful place. You realize that the outcome of your illness is not as important as the outcome of your life, and you spend the time that you have focused on the present. You enjoy the day-to-day events of living. You are awed by the magic and love in those everyday moments. You cease to base your happiness on some far-off future goal. You are pleased just to BE.

PART TWO

THE
GUIDE

Introduction to Part Two

This guide for a successful journey contains a variety of exercises and essays to inspire you and to help you cope with or avoid different kinds of problems. Some of the exercises already have been suggested in Part One to help with specific problems.

You are encouraged to read the entire section first and begin to implement the suggestions. Our hope is that these exercises can be starting points for you to develop your own ideas on how to help yourself. Share the suggestions and your own insights with others close to you.

If you are feeling ill, some of the ideas may require too much energy and effort from you. Pace yourself. Don't expect to do more than one or two activities at one time. Modify activities that don't seem to work for you. The important thing is to keep actively involved in helping yourself.

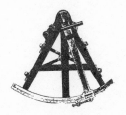

Self

Your self-image is hurt. You are no longer the active, supporting, healthy person you once were—not at this moment. But know that the real you, the inner being that is your essence, is untouched

You still have control over your behavior. You can choose to sail along evenly through the complexities of your body's journey or to fight against them, making yourself and the people you love unhappy.

Ease your mind. Realize that your self-worth comes from your inner being, not your outer self. Your inner being is quiet and subtle and touches the inner beings of others. The activities that flow from your inner being bring love and caring and depth of feeling to those around you. They color your inner world, which is the only "real" world you have. While your body may undergo disconcerting changes—bloating, or loss of weight, body parts, hair, functioning—your inner self, that quiet place within, remains the same.

Feed your inner being with positive thoughts, peaceful images, and kindness. And those "positives" will touch and energize the lives of those around you.

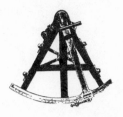

Images

New images—frightening and foreign—surround you. Uniformed strangers with medical paraphernalia enter your life. Your body is theirs to puncture, prod, shave, and cut as they see fit. Uncertainty, lack of control, and apathy throw you off balance, and you feel totally alone.

Rather than attempting to escape your surrounding images, accept them—not in resignation or defeat, but in a participatory way. Become an active part of the scenes you find yourself in.

You are the centerpiece, the focal point, of all this medical activity. You can determine which actions will be taken and which will not. Ask questions. Seek out second and third opinions. Demand answers.

You can choose to see yourself as a victim of your illness, lacking free will, slowly sinking. Or you can choose to see yourself as buoyant, light and flexible, floating on the waters of illness, flowing with the incidents you encounter.

We rarely reflect on the enormous impact our perceptions and images of ourselves and the world around us have on our lives. We are what we imagine ourselves to be.

Use your imagination wisely.

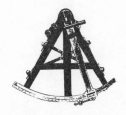

The Unknown

You may come upon frightening times when no one seems to know what is happening to you. While you are the center of much attention, no one has any answers.

You may have three or five or seven physicians "working on your case." Yet no two of them give you the same information. Nurses parry your questions with, "Ask your doctor."

At times like these you will need a deep keel to steady your ship. You yourself are that keel! Deep within you is the strength and steadiness you need. You can discover it if you seek it. You *are* the control! Whatever predictions are made or implied, you have something to say about them. The will to live has overcome statistics more than once. So has the will to die or to let go of life.

Don't get caught in the frantic seas of indecision or fortune-telling. "How long will I live?" "How bad will it get?" "How will it end?" No matter how many answers you gather to these questions, chances are that few, if any, will turn out to be correct.

Steady yourself and focus on *now*.

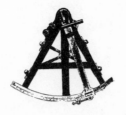

Prayer

Prayer can ease our travel and bring us peace.

Through prayer, we can let go of our burden, pass it along. And we can experience total love and acceptance.

Discover prayers that have special meaning for you, which offer you support and encouragement. Don't punish yourself with guilt left over from the past or disquiet yourself with anxiety for the future. Instead choose to follow the way of peace and goodness in the present.

Write a prayer of your own. Make it personal and complete. Visualize your body as a tiny speck on the earth, and the earth as a tiny speck in the universe. Visualize your spirit as part of the Total Spirit which encompasses all in the universe. Think of your body as a vehicle and your spirit as the living energy that makes it work. Be aware of your spirit's importance and your body's insignificance.

Experience forgiveness and love.

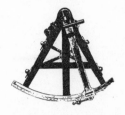

Inner Quiet

I must learn a new way. A peaceful, quiet way to use my energy now. I have been given the challenge to call upon that part of myself which is not dependent on action, that part which taps my spirit and my heart.

I must be the peaceful one. The one who remains in one place as do the mighty trees on my journey's islands. The sun may blister, the winds and storms rage around me, even ripping away parts of my physical being. But I remain solid and still inside.

I absorb the surroundings. I sit in peaceful places with my mind quiet but alert for the depth of life's meaning. It is the way I choose in the quest I have been assigned. I could throw myself overboard, surrendering my freedom, or I could wander without goals or charts through the seas. But I choose to determine the meaning, to find the hidden treasure-places, to expand my awareness.

I accept pain and beauty as two sides of the same seed. And that seed is life.

I will follow my chosen course until I have reached my destination. I will travel with an open heart and a strong will. Like a tree whose leaves dance in the sunlight, I will be moved, but I will not lose that centered feeling—that still, peaceful place within me that offers me the strength I need to endure.

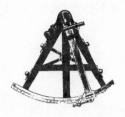

Challenges/Adventure

The American Indians brought up their children in stages. They moved them from their mother's care into adulthood in ritualized periods of recognized growth. Each stage required accomplishment and was symbolized by a new name, new ornaments, new activities. Indian children set goals for themselves and attained these stages at their own pace, by their own actions.

Children of the frontier worked as hard as their parents to survive in the wilderness. They had a sense of contribution. And they too had goals.

But somewhere we have lost our opportunities for adventure in life. We have lost the excitement of exploring, of learning from exploration, of meeting important challenges.

Children today seldom have the chance to test their skills of endurance. Easy living and affluence mean that children's participation is seldom required in activities of importance. They are not called upon to contribute to the family. Nor are they challenged to think as adults. Instead, childhood is a dream world of games and toys.

Suddenly childhood slips away into adolescence. And adolescents' challenges seem to come mainly from their peers. Dare, just for the sake of bravado! Take a drug and escape!

Life has little reality to our children, little meaning to our young adults. We reach adulthood wondering what it is all about.

We need to reacquaint ourselves with those primitive practices of goal-setting and accomplishment, to set personal goals and mark gradual stages of advancement in our challenging situation. Our goals must be realistic, and we must give ourselves plenty of encouragement along the way. We can't expect to be able to jog a mile two weeks after a major operation. But we can hope for that goal within a reasonable time limit, and we can work in stages to reach it.

Examine the feelings of hopelessness, uselessness, and low self-worth that you may be experiencing. Are you setting realistic goals? Are you giving yourself encouragement and credit for what you are doing?

Life is not how long we live, but how fully we live. Even if you are confined to bed, you still can have a rich and fulfilling life through giving to others and through accepting, with grace, what others do for you.

You are fighting for your life! Don't let old patterns of thinking get in your way. Forget about how you used to approach life's problems. You are not the person you used to be.

You have a new journey before you, and you must assess your strongest qualities—courage, kindness, inner peace, love—and gather them in force to accompany you. You have chosen to undertake your journey with stamina, wit, and grace. At the very beginning of your journey you packed your sea trunk with the things you treasured most. Now, in sorting through, you find that only the most important are left. Your spirit has become lean and vital. You are aware not only of the danger of your journey, but of the beauty.

You are entering new stages of accomplishment. Your feeling of success is great when each obstacle is met and overcome. Although you can have no guarantee of what lies ahead, you are willing to sail smoothly along rather than to allow yourself to be overwhelmed.

Yours is a conquering spirit!

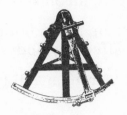

Fear

Your situation can be frightening. Your fears may center around yourself: "Will I be able to cope?" "Will I tolerate pain?" "Will I die?" Or it may concern others: "Will my relatives and friends stand by me?" "Will my doctor abandon me if I refuse a treatment or if I don't get well?" "How will my family deal with my death?"

Fear can paralyze you. It can inhibit your ability to function. It can cause worry, restlessness, and sleeplessness. In turn, these reactions cause your wellness to decay. You become tired, nervous, and irritable.

Fear Exercise

The following exercise will enable you to confront your fear and examine it realistically. Take your time. Don't force yourself to examine too much at one time. Write your responses down here. If you feel too fearful to deal alone with these issues, ask someone close to you to do this exercise with you.

Ask yourself the following questions:

• What is the source of my fear right now? Is it a medical test? A loss? Pain? Death?

- What is the most frightening aspect of my fear?

- If it's a test I fear, am I afraid of the results or of how the test itself may affect my body?

- If it's a loss, do I fear my inability to cope with the loss?

- If it is pain, is it fear that the pain can't be controlled or that I won't be able to cope with it?

- If it is death, is it fear of losing those I love, fear of the unknown, or fear of punishment?

- What realities are my fears founded upon?

- What are the chances that my test results will show that something is wrong?

- What are the chances of my having uncontrolled pain?

- What can I do to alleviate my fear?

Here are some suggestions:

1. Gain more information. Talk over your medical fears with a trusted health professional, a nurse or a doctor. Much of what concerns you may be a remote or nonexistent possibility in your situation, based only on stories you have heard about others' experiences with cancer.

2. Talk over your fears with family, friends, or a counselor. Find someone who can look at the information objectively with you.

3. Talk with someone who knows community resources, like a hospital social worker, a minister, an attorney, or a

financial adviser. Many helpful resources are available. If you don't find help at first, keep trying.

4. Create your own resource list. Include names of persons you can turn to for help, as well as programs and activities which you find most helpful. Consult your list when you feel overwhelmed by your troubles. In such times of stress it's easy to forget your ready sources of help. Keep your resource list in your Captain's Log and add to it.

5. Think of the worst possible scenario and devise plans to alter it. Working on solving issues that can be solved, and learning not to worry about those that cannot be solved, will enable you to look at your fears more realistically.

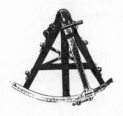

Constructive Denial

A person who has cancer but does not talk about the illness or the possibility of death is said to be in the "denial" phase of the illness.

This comment may be said in a condescending tone, implying that denial is a practice that should be eliminated. But those who have never faced a life-threatening situation have no concept of how the mind works under such circumstances. And those who have faced other kinds of life-threatening situations may not equate them with the experience of cancer.

For instance, many stories have been recounted in the popular media of people who have found themselves in seemingly hopeless predicaments, like this one:

A man fell into a crevice in the snow and was trapped in an underground cavern deep below the surface. He spent his time throwing a heavy object tied to a rope above his head and out through the hole through which he had fallen. He hoped the object would catch between rocks, so that the rope could support his body weight while he climbed to safety. Finally, against great odds, he succeeded—and survived.

This man would be described as clear-headed, courageous, a survivor. Certainly he would not be described as being "in denial" simply because he tried his best to solve this seemingly hopeless situation.

When people are dealing with cancer, however, they are said to be "in denial" if they struggle against the odds. Such thinking implies that it's useless to talk about surviving or to plan for the future when the statistics look grim. This attitude is totally wrong!

Denial becomes a problem only when it is used to escape real problems by avoiding them. Then it needs to be corrected, usually with professional help.

In order for those who are not going through the cancer experience to understand denial, they must first imagine themselves in the same circumstances. If you knew that you had only a few months to live, what would you spend your time thinking about? Would you be able to maintain your constant state of worry and anxiety for that long? Could you contemplate death for that long? Or would you fight to survive against the odds?

It's not how long a person will live, but the quality of her or his remaining days that is important, as the following story bears out:

One man we worked with was given only a few weeks to live. He lived fully for an entire year, long enough to provide for all the needs of his young family. He spent his time working on wellness by exercising, eating well, and practicing positive imagery. His wife said that they had been closer during that time and had made detailed financial preparations for them. He maintained a positive attitude, telling himself and others that he was going to beat the odds.

Some may have worried that he "didn't know how seriously ill he was." But he was just using constructive denial. When denial is used to focus the mind on getting well, it can be one of the most powerful survival tools we have.

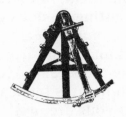

Peace

In the midst of all the chaos, you need to be able to visit a place of peace where you can find strength and renewal. You won't find this place outside yourself, although the "outside" can help you find it. No one but you can give you peace, though others can share theirs with you for a while. You do not have to create this place; it already exists. But, for most of us it has been buried under indifference for years, as we pursued the "outside" aspects of our lives. You don't have to be "religious" to find this peace, although religion is one way to discover it.

What you do need is a belief that inner peace does exist and that you can attain it. To attain peace, you must change the way you think about achieving other goals. You need to recognize that peace is a process.

Many people equate peace with relaxation. Relaxation is fine, but it is a temporary break from activity. Peace is itself an ongoing activity, one that requires your continued involvement.

Most of us are taught to work hard and strive diligently to get what we want. But the quest for peace is different. You can't say, "I'm going to find peace if it kills me." Instead, peace is a letting go of negative thoughts, fears, anxieties, and angers—not fighting them, but simply allowing them to dissolve. In this case, letting go does not mean quitting or giving up. Rather, it is a more effective way of "fighting." If you are at peace, you cannot lose. You realize that there are no guarantees about the physical outcome of your cancer, but your inner peace eliminates fears and anxieties and improves the quality of your life *now*!

You must discover that peaceful place even during bad days. You can become more proficient at finding peace, at allowing your peaceful spirit to be in control.

Peace Exercise

Practice this exercise:

Clear your mind. Repeat a short, uplifting phrase over and over to yourself. Examples: "I choose peace"; "The beauty of life is in me"; "The peace of God is in me—the strength of God surrounds me." If your mind drifts from your phrase—and it *will* wander—do not become discouraged or angry or tense. Simply go back to your phrase. Every time. Peacefully. Away and back, away and back, like a gentle wave lapping on the shore of your consciousness. The more you do this, the more you realize that you can steer your mind and your spirit. You can eliminate the negative things that keep you stuck by letting go of them and allowing yourself to reach your place of peace.

In the grip of pain and discouragement, you can still discover peace and generate peaceful feelings. We have seen many people find peace even in the midst of extreme physical pain.

Open yourself to the possibility of peace, however you perceive it. Peace can conquer anything.

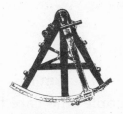

Thinking/Feeling

Feelings are not magical. They do not appear out of nowhere and stay around until they choose to leave!

What you are thinking or telling yourself plays a large role in determining what you feel and how long you'll feel it.

Changing the way you feel is not the same as repressing the way you feel. When you change, you actually feel different. When you repress, you're pretending to yourself and others that you feel different, when actually you do not.

Thinking/Feeling Exercises

If you believe that thoughts and feelings have little in common, try this exercise:

From the following lists, check each thought you have had. Then write down a feeling you had that went along with the thought.

Section A

"Why me?"

"This isn't fair."

"I'll never get better."

"I hate being like this."

"This is terrible."

"My poor family!"

"I'm nothing but a burden!"

Section B

"I'm lucky I have people who care for me."

"I can whip this thing!"

"How can I make the best of this?"

"There are still plenty of things I can do."

"Our family is a team—we love each other."

"Life involves give and take."

"There's nothing wrong with my accepting some help."

If your thoughts tend to mirror those in Section A, your feelings probably are negative—in Section B, probably positive.

Try another thinking/feeling exercise:

Use a blank sheet of paper and write down feelings you have been struggling with lately. Then write down the thoughts you believe are associated with the feelings. Remember, these thoughts are not always obvious or easy to admit. Look carefully, and be honest with yourself. Examples:

Anger: "My doctor makes me mad!"

Sadness: "I miss working and my friends at work."

Depression: "This will only get worse."

Now write down some other feelings that you would like to have and then the thoughts that might bring them about. Examples:

Happiness: "I am getting better!"

Love: "My family is so good to me."

Peace: "I am in God's hands."

These exercises will not seem easy at first, but don't be discouraged. The more you attempt them, the less difficult they will become.

Don't fight negative thoughts. You can't win. It's like someone saying, "Don't think about bananas." And there they are! The only thing you can do is replace negative thoughts with positive thoughts and actions. Actions create their own thoughts, so get involved as actively as you can. Record your progress in your Captain's Log. Make a meal for your family. Read a story to the children. The less you sit and dwell on your problems, the better you will feel. Remember, as long as you are alive, you can make a difference.

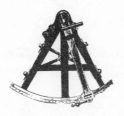

Treatment

"Treatment" can refer to a variety of experiences. It may be radiation therapy, chemotherapy, or surgery. It may be a lymphangiogram, a CT scan, or a barium enema. Many times we're expected to undergo these tests or treatments without knowing anything about them.

Treatment Exercise

This exercise is designed to help you look at these experiences objectively. By examining the reason for the test or treatment—and your feelings about having it—you can be more aware of the significance of the experience and seek help and information if you need it.

Answer the following questions carefully, and write the responses here. You may not feel you need to investigate what is happening to you as fully as this exercise suggests, but make sure you understand how you feel about what you know.

• Do I understand the purpose of this treatment? Why is it being done? Will it provide the doctor with more information about my case? Is it for prevention or early detection of the disease? Is it for control or cure of my illness or for control of pain?

• Do I know what to expect during the treatment? Will I have to drink anything? Will I have an IV? Will I have an injection? Of what?

• What benefits will come from this treatment? Will it ease pain? Will it give information? Will it kill cancer cells?

• What are the negative effects of this treatment? Will there be side effects? What can be done about side effects?

• Will the treatment be painful?

• How do I feel about this procedure or treatment?

• What can I do to improve my feelings about this treatment? Do I understand the benefits? Do I need more information? Do I need a second opinion? Do I need support and reassurance?

Now list what you will do to make this exercise an important and positive one for yourself. Here are some examples:

1. I will remember that the technicians do this job every day. They are competent and careful.

2. I will talk with someone who has had this experience and get that person's perspective.

3. I will not listen to secondhand horror stories without facts to substantiate them.

4. I will remember that staff activities are not always centered on me. A worried look on my doctor's face may be the result of a phone call he received before he entered my room. An instrument being prepared for use may not be for me.

5. Instead of thinking of how bad I will feel during the treatment, I will think of how good I will feel when it is over.

6. I will think of the benefits it will provide for me.

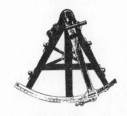

Life/Death

Since cancer is perceived as a life-threatening disease, regardless of how many people are cured of it, the fear of death becomes more real when cancer is diagnosed. Fear of death can overwhelm appreciation of life.

A person who had cancer and who came very close to death once said, "You are alive until you die." This statement sounds simplistic, yet, upon reflection, you'll discover that it has profound meaning. The point is that "dying" is a noncategory. Dying is living with a focus on the final outcome of the experience of life, which is death. This is a limited—and unpleasant—perspective. If, instead, we focus on living, we get the most out of our lives.

In fact, the diagnosis of cancer can provide us with a valuable lesson. It can force us to come to grips with death on a personal level. Death is something we will all experience. If we are able to make peace with death, we will truly appreciate all that we have in our lives, and we will find we can be more relaxed about the diagnosis of cancer.

It's important to remember that many people are cured of their cancer. Even those with advanced cancer have overcome the odds and the prognosis and have survived even after they were told they had just a few months to live.

Cancer does not have to be a death sentence. But it should be an alarm to your psyche.

You need to muster all your inner strength and energy to fight for the kind of life you want, without regard for the amount of time involved. You must be prepared for death in all ways, but then you must turn away from death and live as fully as you are able to live. You must take part in your healing. You must realize the power you have within yourself for inner healing. You must say to yourself, "Let death take care of itself. I will take care of living."

There may be times when you're justified in admitting that you're tired of the fight. You may feel ready to let go of life. But this can be premature. You may be reacting to complete exhaustion from the disease or the treatment or the psychological impact of your cancer. This is a common experience for those who are quite ill from their disease. With proper care and rest, you'll find that you can recover and take up the journey once again.

Then there are times when letting go of life makes sense. Some persons with the disease may face only continued suffering and discomfort. A person with cancer may feel that death would disappoint the family, that they would feel she or he had given up the fight. It's important for family members to let their loved one know that they appreciate the fight. They must also allow that person to leave the pain and suffering behind. The person with cancer may be seeking permission to leave, and sometimes will linger until the family finally has accepted the idea of death. At such times, conversation should be focused on what needs to be said, not on pep talks about keeping up the fight. Conversations about life and the important feelings in life will affirm and strengthen the bond between persons involved. The focus is on living, not dying.

In summary:

1. Be prepared for death, not because of cancer but because we all die.

2. Embrace life. Really live it. It is precious.

3. Remember, cancer is not a death sentence.

4. Take part in your recovery. Enrich your own wellness.

5. You don't have to accept the time limits put upon you if you don't want to. You can fight as long as you choose.

Family members:

1. Affirm your relationships. Focus on what is positive now.

2. Don't force someone to cling to life if he or she doesn't want it anymore.

3. Live in the moment. Love each other *now*.

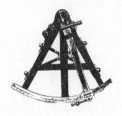

Goals/Accomplishments

In order to set reasonable and realistic goals, and appreciate your accomplishments, here are some specific suggestions:

1. If the comparison depresses you, avoid comparing your current progress to what you used to be able to do as a healthy person. If you used to run three miles a day, walking to your kitchen three times a day probably seems an absurd goal. However, if you haven't walked at all for two weeks, those trips to the kitchen are a major breakthrough!

2. Keep a daily list in your Captain's Log of your accomplishments on that day. This list should be detailed: "Made dinner in thirty minutes"; "Washed my hair with Sue's help"; "Did three leg lifts today." It's important to note what is happening in measurable terms, so you can plot your progress and actually see how you are improving.

3. During a bad day, spend some time focusing on the improvements you have made or on the fact that you will eventually feel happy again.

4. In your Captain's Log, list some long-term physical goals to work toward. It's important to formulate these long-term goals even if you question whether or not you will attain them.

5. Train your mind to look at what is working in your life. Since it's quite obvious what is not working, to concentrate on that serves no one. Keep a record in your Captain's Log of what is working and what you are able to do. You may be surprised at what you can do if you just pay attention to it.

6. When you have a bad day, jot down the events of the day and how you felt about them. You may discover patterns, situations, or people that are not helpful and then decide how to avoid them in the future. Keep this information in your Captain's Log.

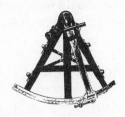

Boredom

We don't always associate boredom with illness, but it is a common feeling. We go from activity, involvement, and productivity to a state of suspended animation. We wonder what to do next. These suggestions will help you pay attention to this aspect of your illness and begin to counteract it:

1. Accept the fact that if you want to stop being bored you're going to have to do something.

2. Write down a list of the ways you have spent your days lately, recording the length of time for each activity. List the names of persons you spent time with.

3. On a scale from one to ten (least to most), rate the pleasure these activities and people bring you. Take a good look at those ratings. Plan how you can spend more time with those people and in those activities that you rate highest.

4. Write down what you used to do for pleasure and satisfaction. Is there any part of this that you can still do?

5. What else can you do? Before you say, "Nothing," write a list of your skills, even if you haven't used them recently.

Determine which of these skills you can use even if you have physical limitations. Get ideas from others.

6. Ask yourself what is stopping you from doing something useful or stimulating. How much of the obstacle comes from the disease? How much from your attitude? Remember, this exercise is to help those who are struggling with boredom. If you're happy with what you're doing, keep it up.

7. Brainstorm with family or friends. Come up with some unusual things for you to do, alone or with others.

8. Make one day's schedule as tight as you can, and leave another day as unstructured as possible. See which one works best for you.

9. Break your routine. Routine can help to anchor you at times. But it can also be deadening.

10. Find some humorous films, tapes, or books. Laughter helps dissolve boredom.

11. DO IT (whatever IT is)! Even though you don't feel that excited about IT. The good feelings will come. Remember, breaking out of boredom can be like cracking through cement.

12. Do something loving for someone. Send a card or a note or a poem. Make a call.

13. Surprise someone. Surprise yourself.

14. Pick up some art supplies—and CREATE! If you say, "I'm just not creative," ask a family member to bring you an *Anti-coloring Book* or two from a bookstore. They stimulate imagination and creativity.

15. Do some things you never had time for when you were more active. Read. Listen to entire symphonies. Sort out toolboxes, sewing cabinets, photos for albums.

16. Remember, if you're bored a lot, you're probably also boring. Enjoy! Let people enjoy you! You can—even with cancer.

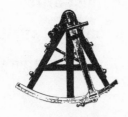

Self-Help

Here is a quick checklist of ways to help yourself. Use it when you feel yourself getting into a negative frame of mind. It will help turn you toward more positive thinking.

1. Keep your thoughts as positive as possible. That doesn't mean you should deny what is happening or hide behind cliches like, "It'll be all right." It means you should look for ways to help yourself.

2. Break your routine.

3. If you're having trouble reading, listen to tapes or records.

4. Listen to music.

5. If you hear songs that uplift you, tape them and create your own collection.

6. Listen for humor. Laugh.

7. Stay involved in activities if you can.

8. Talk with people. Share your ideas and feelings. Get involved with a support group. Set realistic goals and monitor your progress faithfully.

9. Plan your days. Don't just drift.

10. But leave room for spontaneity.

11. Make sure you stay loving—actively.

12. Meditate.

13. Pray.

14. Read through this book again.

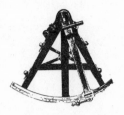

Visualization

We are just beginning to understand the power of our minds, and especially how that power relates to our bodies. Several theories are being tested. But researchers agree on one point: the mind *is* powerful.

Visualization means seeing something in your mind's eye and focusing on it. This can be an image of you sitting on a beach watching a sunset. It can be any image that you find peaceful and relaxing. The key to visualization is that you try to involve all of your senses and put yourself in the picture. Visualization is much more participatory than daydreaming; in a daydream you merely *wish* you were watching a sunset. In visualization, you use your mind to come as close as possible to really experiencing yourself on that warm sand beach seeing that sunset, awed by its beauty.

A special type of visualization was developed by Carl Simonton, M.D., and presented in the book he co-authored with Stephanie Simonton, *Getting Well Again.* This visualization produces a mental image of the cancer and of the forces fighting the cancer, including radiation, chemotherapy, and your body's own immune system. The important intention is that you spend time thinking of the cancer cells in your body as weak and easily defeated. This technique enables you to see your own mental power as a powerful tool at your command. As an aid to visualization, you're encouraged to draw pictures of the images.

Visualization Exercises

Here are some exercises that can help you feel involved in your own recovery. Doing these exercises, while it obviously does not guarantee physical cure, can provide a constructive alternative to depression or boredom.

1. Spend time each day visualizing. Focus on the site of your cancer and imagine the cancer shrinking.

2. Draw your images on paper. Make them as realistic as you can.

3. Use relaxation tapes to guide your images.

4. Keep a peaceful image in your mind, and allow yourself to return to it during quiet times. Use your image when you need to relax or during treatments, while waiting in doctors' offices, before sleep, or when you wake up in the night. The more you practice this exercise, the easier it will be for you to slip into your relaxed image.

5. At first, while you're learning the technique of visualization, don't expect to be able to use it in times of crisis. You must spend time and energy practicing visualization before you can rely on it to counteract negative feelings.

6. Seek out images and relaxation tapes from a variety of sources. Books and tapes are abundant and may be either bought or borrowed. Check your local bookstores and libraries.

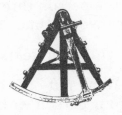

For Family/Friends

As someone close to a person who has cancer, you have special problems and concerns. The following suggestions will help you assess your own needs and cope with your situation.

Above all, have realistic expectations.

One of the biggest obstacles you will face is a feeling of inadequacy because you are unable to make the person well.

1. Be aware of what you *should not expect to do*.

    • You cannot cure the person of cancer. Medical professionals are working on that.

    • You can't always cheer up the person. The person just may not be able to be cheerful right now! Besides, if you only visit with the intent of bringing cheer, you might miss the chance for a real discussion.

    • Your purpose is not simply to distract the person. Television and crossword puzzles do that quite nicely.

2. Be aware of what you *can do*.

    • You can love the person unconditionally. Family and friends are best at that!

• You can support the person through good and bad times—be there for the bad times too.

• You can share laughter and tears.

• You can be real. Don't put on a happy face when you don't feel happy. Your person with cancer already is dealing with a situation that seems unreal; don't compound the unreality. Because people with cancer need ordinary, familiar reality in their lives, treat them as you always have.

Family/Friends Exercise

Make a list of the following things:

1. What you have already done for the person with cancer.

2. What you are willing to do for that person—and what you can do, realistically.

3. How you have made a difference in that person's life—physically, emotionally, and spiritually. If you have trouble with these answers, ask the person with cancer to help you.

Family/Friends: Caring for Yourself

Probably you have put your needs and pleasures aside. It's time to bring them out! You must support yourself if you plan to continue to help others. There is nothing worse—or less effective—than "helping" when you are tired and resentful. You cannot disguise these feelings. So it's much better for everyone concerned if you take care of yourself before you get to this point.

It's normal to have personal needs and to try to meet them. If you give and give and keep on giving, without replenishing yourself, you will quickly become depleted. The most important thing about you for the person with cancer is *you*. Just your presence—whether you're there physically or in spirit—is what matters.

Don't put pressures on yourself when you don't need to. Just be loving, warm, angry, scared, happy, sad, real—YOU.

Here are more suggestions:

1. Write down your personal needs for each day, just the basic things you do for yourself, like washing your hair, taking a shower, going for a walk—whatever you do in your routine daily activities.

Check your list and make sure you do these things every day.

You may want to time these activities to see how little time they take. When you are dealing with a difficult problem in your life, even the simplest activities seem to take forever, when actually they are accomplished in minutes.

2. Make a list of pleasant activities you enjoy. It may be seeing movies, eating out, playing tennis—anything that enables you to get away from the immediacy of the problem and relax.

Make sure you have time to do at least one of these things weekly. Guilt feelings about leaving the person alone when he or she is unable to get out should be countered by the picture of yourself as the caretaker later in the week, exhausted and emotionally strung out.

Helping in the Hospital

A person with cancer in the hospital, for whom the world is defined by walls and corridors, especially needs to keep in touch with his or her identity and personal lifestyle. As a friend or family member, you are in a prime position to be of help in keeping that person linked to the real world. You can bring in accounts of the everyday, normal moments that the hospitalized person is missing.

Many family members avoid talking about day-to-day normalities for fear of depressing their loved one who can't be home. Actually, hearing about and being involved in "outside" events helps hospitalized individuals keep their perspective and sanity.

What's more important, these links help them remember their role in life and provide a tangible goal to work for.

Here are some suggestions:

1. If the person feels like eating, bring in a treat from a favorite restaurant.

2. Bring in some LIFE—kids, plants, goldfish.

3. Bring in a tape player. Provide tapes of music, lectures, sermons, family gatherings, or everyday activities like dinner conversations or the kids' bedtime. Leave the tapes there to be played when you're not there.

4. Bring in articles on topics of interest to the person. Read aloud.

5. If possible, take the person out on a leave—for a picnic, a movie, or a haircut.

PART THREE

CAPTAIN'S
LOG

Introduction to Part Three

This section is a guide for journal-keeping. It provides a format and a sample page to get you started on recording your experiences and insights on your voyage. Use the questions here and record your answers in a separate notebook. You may want to answer the questions in Part Two in this same notebook.

Keeping a log requires discipline and perseverance. If you allow yourself time to work on it, it can help you sort through the emotions—stormy and passive—that threaten to sink you at times. Also, you'll be able to look back over your entries and note your growth and progress. Your journal is your personal record. You may choose whether or not to share it with others.

If you write consistently in your Captain's Log, you'll find it easier every day. Get a sturdy notebook, so you won't lose any valuable material. And begin.

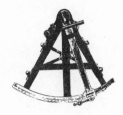

Captain's Log: A Model

Sample Questions

Date and time:

1. What did you experience today?

2. How did you feel about your experience?

3. What did you do about your feelings?

4. What good things happened today?

5. In what ways did you grow today?

6. In what ways did you show love for someone today?

7. How did others show they love you?

8. What good conversations did you have today? With whom? About what?

9. What new ideas did you have today?

10. What did you learn today?

These are suggestions. Use the questions you find useful. Or devise your own.

PART FOUR

PEACE SUPPLIES

Introduction to Part Four

At times during your journey you'll find that a simple thought with a single idea will be the greatest help to you. For those moments of intensity and concern or quiet reflection, here are Peace Supplies, thoughts capsulized in brief phrases for you to ponder. Sit quietly and allow your mind to stay with each one for a time as you contemplate its meaning.

You may use this section for meditation, using a well-loved phrase for a mantra. You may wish to copy your favorites and tape them to your mirror or your desk or any other place that you pass by regularly, so that they can feed your spirit. From these slogans and phrases, you may be inspired to create your own. Or you may want to illustrate with drawings or paintings or photographs the images these phrases bring to mind.

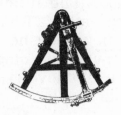

Affirmations

Love is strength.
Love is healing.

I will live today to the fullest I can.
If every day is lived that way, I will have done what I can do.

The peace of God is in me.
The strength of God surrounds me.

Sometimes it is difficult to accept help.
I feel like a burden.
But I must trust in the process of love and life.
I am learning and growing as I accept help, because it is
    time for me to learn about acceptance.
Others are learning and growing from giving, because it is
    time for them to give.
In essence, I am giving while I am receiving.

I accept the fact that I am afraid at times.
Fear is not an enemy, but rather a friend
    whom I allow in, with graciousness and love,
    only to find that it must leave quickly
    because the brightness of love
    is more than fear can handle.

    It is said that all life comes from the sea.
    We equate life with the sea.
    When we are alive we are immersed in the sea of life.
    We float and drift and dive in the waves of living.

Illness strikes, and we are tossed and tumbled into the surf.
Torments of illness and fear take control of our bodies.
Finally, we lie beached upon the sand.
Perhaps the sea barely laps at our feet.
Perhaps the ghost crabs of death whisper in our ears.

We must gently push ourselves to wade back into life.
We must overcome the surf, dive through the breakers
    of illness which try again to smash us onto the beach.
We must immerse ourselves once more in the tides
    and flow of living.

Wash the illness from your body, in a gentle yet forceful
    flow away from you.
Energy flows from deep within the spirit, filling the void
    with a clean, golden warmth.
Love the energy. It radiates to all parts of your body and
    mind.
Love of self, love of others, love of the infinite, love of God,
Natural state of being, that which is meant to be,
Eases the feelings, the soul into a calm, smooth place,
Sustaining life, love, relationships, sharing,
Sustaining self, not only the physical self, but the self for
    which we are loved, cared for, and admired.

Purifying your spirit with the knowledge of your goodness,
Easing fear, anger, guilt, and other negative thoughts from
    your awareness,
Allowing the strength and energy of life to flow into your
    being,
Caring, warmth, and prayers lift your tired body upon them,
Elevating your spirit above the mundane and bathing you in
    the golden world of peace.

Respect yourself. Give yourself credit for the kind and
    helpful human being you are. Recognize your ability
    to love and care for others and to love yourself.

Energize your inner being. Focus on your heart. Travel
    throughout your entire being slowly and completely.
    Liquify your physical being.

Let your feelings of strain and stress ooze from you until
    your body is limp.

Accept the fact that you cannot alter the entire world, that
    this world undergoes continuous change and you will
    never "get ahead" of it.

Accept yourself as part of that ongoing process of change
    and growth.

Visualize your thoughts as X-rays, images in muted grays,
    barely recognizable, so that your mind is unable to focus
    on any sharp or distinct form.

Life, teeming, full of gentle motion, overflowing.
High energy emanates from within.
Volumes of words attempt to grasp the undefinable
    essence of the spirit which alights in the body until
    time to depart.

                                        I choose peace.

Being, oneness, captured in the physical world,
Eluding time, definition, limits,
    it dwells in a space all its own,
Always seeking awareness of its presence—a glimpse
    of a wildflower just off the path,
Uplifting the burdened spirit,
    pulling the soul above itself,
    opening to all who are willing to see,
Tempting us to the infinite, the place where beauty lies.
You may succumb to its temptation,
    accept its precious gift.

May the beauty of life fill me with joy.

Although I have sickness in me,
I also have wellness in me.
I will focus on the wellness,
    and allow it to overcome the sickness.

I am health.
I am wellness.

My spirit moves my body.
My spirit is healthy.
My spirit is alive.

I will gather strength from peace.
From the peace of my soul will come the power of healing.

When the body is out of harmony, it becomes ill.
I will focus on putting my body back in harmony.

I am part of the universal consciousness.
I will open myself to the wisdom and strength
    that resides in the universe.

This moment is precious.
I will not waste it.

I am worthwhile.
I have dignity.
The beauty of God is in me.

The future is but a thought.
The past is but a thought.
The present can become lost in these thoughts
    or enriched by them.
I choose enrichment.

I will trust my sense of myself.
When I am tired I will rest.
When I am energized I will act.
But through all of this I will be.

Death is part of life.
I can accept death and still fight to live.

When I hurt in the present, I at least have something
    I can contend with.
When I fear the future, I make myself helpless.
The future is out of my power. The present is not.

Becoming aware of the possibility of death
    has its good points.
It makes me aware of limits.
It makes me know I must get on with my life now.

When I trust in myself, I am at peace.

When I feel the presence of love in my soul,
I am in touch with God
    and a sense of life that far transcends
    what I am aware of now.

I learn every day,
    except when I spend my time
    wishing today was different.
Then I just mark time.

        I love.
        I live.

            I will not wait to be cured.
            I will participate in the process of wellness.

There are times when I am almost overwhelmed
    by loneliness.
Even with the people who care about me,
    I sometimes feel alone and isolated.

At those moments I need to understand that
    what I am experiencing might not be loneliness,
    but aloneness—the awareness that even the people
    who love me most cannot enter my experience totally.

At those moments of awareness I am open to the more subtle
    recognition of a force or Power or entity
    that joins me in my aloneness,
    a force that seems to be saying,
    "Allow your a/loneness to change to at/oneness."

I will LIVE for as long as I am alive.

Sometimes I become frightened when I think of death.
There are so many unknowns...so many questions...
    leaving others behind...unfinished business...
    unfulfilled dreams.
But then I realize that I am still alive.
And every moment is a new chance.

Serenity is mine.

PART FIVE

YOUR PERSONAL SUPPORT GROUP

Introduction to Part Five

Consider this dialogue among members of a cancer support group as your personal support group. The group members here are composites of cancer patients the authors have worked with in recent years. The problems they struggle to cope with and express are true to life. A variety of problems and suggestions are presented in a support group setting, and you can learn a great deal by listening to how others have dealt with situations similar to yours. Ultimately, of course, your solutions must come from within you. You will hear no final answers, just possibilities.

Here are short descriptions of the "people" in this model group—which includes those with cancer, as well as family members. They are not intended to portray real persons, but to represent typical problems and solutions that arise from the actual experiences of people with cancer and their families. Obviously every possible situation and type of cancer cannot be represented. If your situation differs drastically from those presented here, you can still learn by looking for ideas to help yourself.

Investigate the possibility of attending a support group in your area.

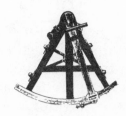

Personal Stories

MARY

Mary is a seventy-five-year-old widow with no children. She discovered she had ovarian cancer five months ago, and after surgical removal of the tumor, she began a series of chemotherapy treatments. Her treatments are very aggressive; each time a treatment is scheduled, she has a hard time forcing herself to keep the appointment. She is uncomfortable expressing herself, and she is increasingly depressed.

ANN

Ann and Hank, in their late twenties, have been married for five years and have a two-year-old daughter. Hank is receiving radiation therapy for Hodgkin's disease. The strain of dealing with Hank's illness, along with financial pressures and the demands of a toddler, have created tensions between them. Ann sometimes wonders why she has a husband who is so ill when her friends are living carefree, "normal" lives.

LOU

Lou, now sixty, has been married for forty years to Marie. Marie, at fifty-nine, is dying of breast cancer which has spread to her bones. In the twelve years since her cancer was diagnosed, she has had surgery, radiation, and chemotherapy. The couple have discussed their situation many times and feel that they have come to accept Marie's condition. They hope that Marie will continue to have good pain control and that she will not lose the limited mobility she still has.

SAM

Sam's fourteen-year-old son, Justin, just learned that he has leukemia. Justin is doing well with chemotherapy, but Sam's wife, Lisa, can think of nothing but losing her child. She blames herself for not noticing the symptoms earlier. Sam is trying to be strong and supportive for both of his loved ones. He tries to overcome his fears and anxieties with positive thinking. But he is concerned that Lisa's behavior will upset his son. He is uncertain of how to help his son, as well as his wife.

HELEN

Helen, aged thirty-five, has never smoked and was shocked when, after a long bout with pneumonia, her doctor put her in the hospital and discovered that she has lung cancer. Her doctor has told her she has eighteen months to live. She is angry. She is also concerned about how her husband, John, and three young children, who are aware of her illness but not of the prognosis, will react to the news. She has always been the "strong one" in the family and is now resentful because she feels she won't get much support from her husband.

JOE

Joe is forty-nine. He was diagnosed with cancer of the colon a year ago. He has a colostomy, which he has adjusted to fairly well. He is divorced and has little contact with his family. His disease is in remission, and he hopes for a cure. But he is angry about the treatment he received from the medical staff; he felt that no one took the time to explain his situation to him.

SUE

At thirty-four, Sue recently has had a lump removed from her breast and radiation therapy to the area. Although she did not have a mastectomy, she is dealing with her altered body image. She wonders if she will ever meet a man who will want to marry a "cancer patient." She also wonders if she should even consider having children.

BOB

Bob, at fifty-three, is a successful businessman. When he coughed up blood one morning, he reminded himself that he needed to cut down on the cigarettes. The second time it happened, a sense of dread came over him. He knew his diagnosis before the initial test results confirmed that he had cancer. After the initial shock wore off, he decided to approach his cancer as he would any business problem. His wife, Fran, is supportive and hopes that he will slow down and enjoy his life with her.

SCOTT AND JUDY

Scott and Judy are the group facilitators.

147

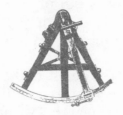

Helplessness

SCOTT: What was the toughest thing you had to deal with when you found you had cancer?

BOB: Well, for me it was a helpless feeling. I went from a life where I felt like I was on top of things to—I don't know what you'd call it—maybe chaos. Everything was out of whack. People were telling me where to be, what to do. I was getting stuff pumped into my body. I guess it was the idea that my life wasn't my own anymore.

SUE: I can relate to that. You know, when I found out I had breast cancer I was so shocked that in some ways it didn't even sink in. Cancer was a word, a terrifying word, but something I didn't have any experience with. You just never think it will happen to you. But when I went in the hospital, then it really started to get through. I was scared and I felt really helpless. In fact, to be honest, I felt like a number, not a human being. It wasn't because the doctors or nurses were nasty or anything like that. In a way I bought being a number because numbers don't have any feelings.

HELEN: I guess my helplessness centered around the idea that my body wasn't doing what it was supposed to do.

It was out of control. I was out of control. God, I can remember not knowing what to do, where to turn, who to trust—and then wondering if it even made any difference.

BOB: Yeah. That idea of "does it make any difference anyway" almost sank me. I started doing nothing but watching TV—and I never watch TV. In fact, I really wasn't paying attention, just sort of staring at it. I couldn't even tell you what was on. It just kept me from thinking about the fact that I have cancer.

SUE: I felt almost paralyzed. I didn't know what to do. Part of me didn't think that what I did made a difference, and yet part of me was scared to death of making the wrong decisions. Especially since I decided not to have a mastectomy. Everyone told me how lucky I was not to lose my breast. I kept wondering how I can be so lucky when I have cancer!

SCOTT: What did you do to combat these feelings of helplessness and move past them?

HELEN: I'm not sure you ever totally work past the feeling. I still have flashes of the old helplessness, especially when I have a bad day. But it doesn't last as long as it used to. What I try to do—and I'm not always successful—is to tell myself that there are lots of things I'm not in control of that don't make me feel helpless. Like an earthquake could hit, or an accident, but it doesn't do any good to dwell on it. I told myself I was tired of being helpless. I did not like the feeling. I still get it sometimes though. I guess I always will. But it isn't going to run my life.

SUE: I looked around and said—literally said—to myself, This is nuts. Here I was, worrying about dying and then wasting my life with all these negative feelings. It was like if I only had a short period of time to live, I owed it to myself to use it wisely. Now that I feel I have a chance for a normal life span, I still realize that I owe myself and others the best life I can make.

BOB: I really got scared and I had somebody talk to me, a counselor. She told me that if I was concerned about being helpless, I needed to get back in touch with the things in my life that I could control. My first thought was my job. I had power and control there, but now that didn't seem to matter. Then I realized I had really lost touch with my family, and I began to work on regaining a relationship with them. I felt I had control of my own choices and that I'd made a good one and had something important to work toward.

JOE: I'll tell you what I did. I got mad. I started asking more questions. I didn't just lie back and let the medical team do what they wanted. At first I was a little nervous that they might get mad at me, and who wants their doctors and nurses mad at them? But then I thought, "It's my body," and even though they might know more about what makes me tick, it still is my body and I've got some say in what happens to it. And, you know, I started feeling better. I started feeling like I was doing something for myself.

ANN: I don't have cancer. My husband does. But what helped us a lot was just coming to this support group. I'll tell you, it was really an eye-opener for me—finding other people who were going through the same thing. All of a sudden I, and my husband too, didn't feel so alone or as helpless because here were a lot of people who were doing something about their cancer.

LOU: Our religion is important to my wife and me. I realized that I had to turn things over to God and let Him help me. As soon as I did that, I felt better. I felt support.

SCOTT: What you are all saying in different ways is that you are only helpless as long as you think of yourselves as helpless. As soon as you do something about it, you feel better.

BOB: I don't think what you do is as important as just the fact that you are doing *something*. You're getting involved. If you're involved, you aren't helpless.

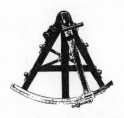

Anger

JUDY: Let's talk about anger. When did you first feel angry?

HELEN: I first felt angry when I heard I had cancer. I looked upward and shook my fist and said, Why me, God? I looked round me at people who were HEALTHY. I mean they had no major problems, and there they sat—smoking! Abusing themselves! I had three kids, and there were old people or bums healthy as horses and I never smoked and I had cancer!

JOE: I didn't get angry at God. My anger was—and still is—directed at my physicians. They are only interested in how much money they'll make, not in me as a person! There was a time I was waiting to hear the results of my test. I was so anxious I couldn't eat or sleep. I had to wait for a whole week when I knew the results were there the very next day. I called the office, but the doctor was out of town, and the receptionist couldn't give me the results over the phone. I was so angry I slammed the telephone in her ear!

SUE: I remember a time when I was furious because I had to have those tattoos for radiation therapy. Even though I had a scar from my surgery, I focused on the tattoos as just one more insult to my body. It didn't matter that it didn't make sense—I just didn't want them!

BOB: When I got down as low as I could go and the doctors told me I could have as little as six months to live, I got mad. I thought, Who do you think you are to tell me that? You're not God. I'll prove you wrong. And I have!

JUDY: So you turned your anger into a positive thing, an energy force that you could draw on for strength to overcome the cancer?

BOB: Yes. When I felt down and really miserable, I would remember that angry feeling and it helped me push myself into doing what I wanted to do.

HELEN: I know what you mean. There were times when I could barely get out of bed, barely get to the bathroom and back, but I pushed myself. Each day I tried to do a little more and I kept a record of how I was doing. On a day-to-day basis I didn't feel like I was making any progress, but when I checked my record I could see I had accomplished much more than, say, two weeks before. I think we can all do better if we can see some progress, no matter how small it is.

SUE: I remember one day I came storming into the house, really angry. I wasn't making any sense. I had so much anger in me I didn't know what to do with it. It wasn't focused on anything, really. I was upset that I had cancer and that I had to have radiation. I was only in my thirties and I was too young for all that. My dog took one look at me, put his tail between his legs and ran! I just burst out laughing. Then I cried. Then I laughed again.

JOE: When I got angry, I had to work. I would do something simple, like sorting out a junk drawer, you know, where you throw everything. If I felt better, I'd go outdoors and mow the lawn, in fifteen-minute parcels, or I'd garden for fifteen

minutes. Being physically and mentally occupied helped me.
I couldn't really change what I was angry about. I have
cancer and nothing will change that, but, like Bob, I used that
energy to motivate me.

SUE: Sometimes I'd be really terrible to my family. They
were trying so hard to help me, but I couldn't be pleased.
I complained—really acted like a spoiled brat. I feel bad
about it now. It was like I knew they'd be there for me.
They really stood by me. Once in a while my brother would
tell me off. He'd tell me he loved me and he understood why
I was behaving like a child but that he wasn't going to put up
with it just because I had cancer.

LOU: When my wife was angry, I was very hurt and upset.
I didn't know how to please her, to cheer her up. She'd snap
at everything I tried to do. Then I talked it over with my
priest, who explained that she really was angry at the cancer
and her loss of her health. He told me to let the anger just
pass through me, not to attach any significance to it or to let
it hurt me. I've been doing much better now, even though it
is still hard.

ANN: I was very angry at my husband for getting sick! It took
me a while to figure it out. I acted like a sweet and dutiful
wife while I was helping him, but I was boiling inside. I was
upset because all my friends had normal, happy lives. They
had plenty of money. And I was stuck with a sick, tired, weak
husband who couldn't even earn a living! One day he asked
for a drink of water. I had just sat down, and I was
exhausted. I slammed the glass down, and then began to cry.
We had a heart-to-heart talk. We had been so busy trying to
take care of each other we just hadn't been open about our
feelings. He understood how I felt and made me realize it
was normal. He helped me. It made him feel better too.

SCOTT: What I'm hearing is that the best way you all have found to deal with your anger is to use the energy from the anger in a positive way. Use it to motivate yourself.

HELEN: That's easier said than done.

ANN: True. But I don't want to spend my life being angry.

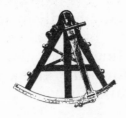

Communication

LOU: Marie and I have a good relationship because we've worked at it and learned over the years how to stay close, even when we are both stressed. Oh, we still have our problems like most people, but we've learned that you've got to talk them through.

SUE: I think it's wonderful. But it's sure the opposite of what happened to me. When I was in the hospital, my parents acted like they never heard of cancer. We were like strangers. I became very guarded in what I said because I didn't want to scare them off any further than they already were.

SAM: Everybody's being cheerful, but nobody's meaning it. I know. When we would visit Justin, you would have thought we didn't know each other. It was like we were at a party making small talk.

LOU: I know. We've seen it a lot in the hospital rooms we've been in with other people. One lady said she felt so alone, even though she had lots of family visiting. Her family acted as though everything would be just the same as it was before. But it never will be.

ANN: Well, sometimes the breakdown comes from the patient's side. My husband hardly ever talks to me about the cancer and how he is feeling. He always just says he's fine and everything will be fine and to just think positively. Sometimes I get sick of hearing "think positive." Don't get me wrong. I know it works for you. But sometimes they are just empty words.

BOB: I agree with you, Ann. Thinking positive is important, but you can't ignore everything else that's going on, or use the phrase to dismiss somebody. That's what it sounds like to me—he's just sort of dismissing you.

ANN: He is! Maybe he's trying to protect me. But I don't want to be protected! I want to know what's going on. I want him to share with me what he's going through so that I can be of some help to him. Even if it's just listening.

SUE: Ann, have you told him how *you* feel?

ANN: Well, sort of. I start feeling like an interrogator. I keep asking him questions about different things.

SUE: But do you tell him how you feel?

ANN: He just says, "Don't worry, it'll be all right." I don't want to upset him, so I just shut up.

BOB: But you're miserable inside.

LOU: I think you've got to tell him what's going on with you.

SUE: Don't get mad at him or try to make him feel guilty. Tell him what you want to say, and how the way you've been talking and interacting just hasn't been working for you.

SAM: I do the same thing, Ann. I hold stuff inside and then get upset if people can't figure it out. But lately, especially with my son, I've been really making an effort to communicate with him. It's really hard, but I think it's paying off. At first it seemed strange because I just didn't talk to him about certain things. I didn't think it was right for a parent to discuss how he felt with his child. But now that Justin realizes I am for real, we have no problems opening up to each other.

JOE: When my kids came to see me the first time, they started this sort of phony pep talk, like cheerleaders. You know: "Hang in there!" "You can do it!" "Rah, rah, rah!" I told them to knock it off! We never talked like that before, and we weren't going to start now!

BOB: Yeah, Joe, I think that's a good point. You should try to be consistent with the way you communicated in the past. Cancer doesn't make you a visitor from another planet!

SAM: That's true to a degree, Bob. But if the way you talked in the past was not very good, this is a real good time to get things turned around.

SUE: That's right. That's what I told myself. There isn't time for these silly games. Even though my cancer is gone and I'm doing pretty well, I still appreciate that we don't necessarily have the time we think we do.

BOB: A sort of "let's get on with it" attitude.

SUE: Yes, exactly.

HELEN: I agree. Even though I struggle with this depression, I really do believe that time is precious and I've got to use it as effectively as I can.

LOU: And don't forget God, or whatever you call your Higher Power. I've gotten an incredible amount of strength and wisdom from praying.

BOB: Interestingly enough, I get the same thing from meditation, which I guess is pretty much like prayer. Sort of a letting go and trusting that there are things we don't understand, but that somewhere it makes sense.

MARY: I have trouble relaxing and letting go. Like I said before, my mind just keeps tuning in on negative thoughts.

LOU: That's why prayer is so helpful. You're asking God to share your burden. If you let Him, you can really take the pressure off yourself.

MARY: I guess I'm not really religious.

BOB: You don't have to be—quote—religious—unquote. People do all sorts of different things—like praying to a traditional God or maybe their own idea of God or a Higher Power. They also ask for help from people in their cancer support group or in their family. What they are saying basically is, "I can't do this alone. I would like some help."

SUE: And that doesn't make you weak or helpless.

SAM: You know, maybe if I wasn't so judgmental about how my wife can't handle the situation with our son better...."

MARY: You mean his cancer.

SAM: Yes, his cancer. I guess I still have trouble saying the word, don't I? But if I got off her back with my expectations and talked to her about my feelings, maybe things would be better. I keep trying to change her attitude instead of accepting her the way she is.

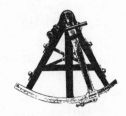

Spirituality

JUDY: How about your spiritual life. How did the cancer help you or disturb you?

SAM: Disturb is the word! I'm still angry at God, if there is one. I don't understand why my son had to be the one to get sick. He's an innocent child. And my poor wife has just lost control. She's unable to function, she's so full of grief and worry.

ANN: I was taught that you can't be angry at God. He isn't at fault. If you pray and believe, you'll be healed. I was told to have faith that my husband will recover and he will, and that the Lord has given us this burden to carry so that we'll become better people. I was told that it isn't punishment, but in a way it's a gift. I'm not that good! Maybe it is a gift, but I'm having trouble accepting that!

LOU: Marie and I have a deep faith. We don't look for answers or reasons why this has hit us. We simply ask for courage and strength to deal with it. At first it was hard to understand, but now we have lived with it and thought about it for a lot of years. It's not easy, but we've found real peace in our faith. I guess we've accepted things the way they are.

HELEN: I guess I'm not a religious person, but I am a spiritual person. I feel there is a deep spiritual power inside of me that guides me. I think it's helping me get through this part of my life. I guess I'm still looking for an answer. John uses his faith to deny what's going on with me. He believes that it's God's will and that, whatever happens, God will help us deal with it. That's fine for him, but it's my life we're talking about!

BOB: Maybe he's right, Helen. I believe in God and I believe in me. I know I'll lick this thing just as I've done in the past. Whenever I have a seemingly insurmountable problem, I work hard on it until I master it. I think I need to play a role with God and with my physicians to help me improve my chances.

HELEN: I agree with you, Bob. That's right. That's a fine way of believing, but I'm saying that John will not even admit that I might die. It's not like I have a magic wand and can make it all go away. I don't want to die, but I have to think of what needs to be done if I do. I'll fight as hard as I can, and I have a positive attitude in spite of the odds. If I die, I just want to know that things will be taken care of as I want them to be. John just can't deal with that, and it worries me. I wonder how he'll do if I die. He doesn't realize how seriously ill I am.

BOB: I guess I don't have to worry about anything that happens once I'm gone, but I can see your point, Helen.

LOU: Marie and I have all our arrangements made. We did that several years ago. It's just a chore that needs to be done, no matter what your state of health is. In a way, it's a gift to be able to make those arrangements, to give them some thought, to have time to say good-bye to people you care about. I know Marie has made a special effort to do something nice for all of our children and grandchildren, something special for them to remember her by.

JUDY: Maybe if John can't bring himself to those preparations, you can accomplish them yourself, Helen. I think it's important that you be honest about your feelings. Tell him what you are doing and why. If he can't deal with it, he might shut you out, but at least you will have tried. And it may open a new channel of communication for the two of you.

SUE: I think it's odd that we've switched our conversation away from our spiritual relationships with God or whatever and are talking about issues surrounding death. It's probably because we can't think about having cancer without thinking about death, and that makes us think about our relationship with God. I find that I get a good feeling from thinking about God. I can turn my troubles over to Him and feel secure that He will help me. I don't expect Him to cure me, just to help me get through, whatever the outcome is.

JUDY: Yes, Sue. There are different aspects to this conversation. One is our relationship with death and the practical aspects of death. The other is our relationship with God. What I'm picking up from all of you is that the spiritual side is a personal and meaningful one for each of you—yet it's different for each of you too. You're saying that your spiritual side helps you get in touch with the issues surrounding death and as a source of peace. It is important to explore this area for yourselves.

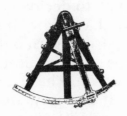

Depression

SCOTT: What other feelings have you experienced? What else have you dealt with or are you dealing with right now?

HELEN: Well, I'll tell you what I'm still struggling with—and that's depression. I have lung cancer and I know what the stats are for lung cancer.

MARY: They're not good, are they?

HELEN: You're not kidding! Every time I think about it I get more depressed. I've got three young kids who need their mother, and I'm probably not going to be here for them. In fact, I'm just about useless right now with my treatments and being so tired all the time. *(She begins to cry softly.)*

BOB *(gently):* Helen...aren't you giving up a little prematurely? I've got lung cancer too. In fact, I've had bone "mets," which you don't have, and I know the stats are not promising. But I still think I can beat this thing. In fact, I know I can beat it. One thing I know for sure is that I can't sit around being depressed all the time.

MARY: That's not so easy—to decide not to be depressed, Bob. I'm seventy-five, and a widow. It seems like one thing after another! I'm just getting worn out. I never expected that my old age would be such a painful time for me. I always thought that we would have a wonderful retirement. But it just didn't work out that way, and now all I have to look forward to is pain and suffering.

JOE: Mary, I know what you're talking about. I'm divorced. I have cancer of the colon and I have a colostomy. I started to look around and say, What else can happen? I found out. I really hit bottom. The world didn't look gray; it looked black! Then I was in the hospital for a while with a man who was a lot worse off than me. He was right at the end and he knew it, but you wouldn't believe his attitude! He was helping me feel better! He'd ask how I was doing and how my boys were. He'd always tell me how lucky I was to have two grown boys who weren't embarrassed to tell their father they loved him. You know, I hadn't even paid attention to that. I asked him how he stayed so positive when he was so sick. He said he could spend his remaining time—however long that might be—being negative or being positive. He said it just didn't make sense to him to be negative; it wouldn't change anything. And he kept that positive outlook.

SUE: I think what helped me was—I started to see that when I was depressed I was constantly thinking about me and how awful it was that I had breast cancer at only thirty-four and that no man would want to marry me since I was "damaged goods." I had always planned for things—my career, marriage, children. When I got cancer, I didn't think I wanted to have children anymore. The risk was too great for them and for me. Then I began to see that there were people who cared for me no matter what happened to me physically. There were people I could care for, people I could give to. Those people helped me believe in the power of love and of hope. I quit dwelling on me and how bad it was.

HELEN: I don't mean to sound obnoxious, Sue. I just can't help but think that you don't have three kids who might be left without a mother.

SUE: That's just it, Helen. You're spending your energy on what might happen, and I underline *might*. You're not paying attention to the fact that you're still alive and have all kinds of opportunities to be with your kids and love them and be loved by them. Don't miss *now.* Don't spoil what you can have by thinking about what may happen.

BOB: That's where I'm at. Every moment is special. Sure, some of the time I'm physically sick and I don't feel like doing anything, but I try to squeeze as much life out of every minute I can. I don't know how to say this, but, even though I know I'm going to beat this cancer, the whole idea of death being real has made me appreciate getting involved in my life...especially *giving.* I enjoy doing things for people—even little things like a card or a phone call. It helps me as much as them because I feel good when I do it.

LOU: When we found out about my wife's cancer, we decided to do some things we had been putting off, and we feel pretty good about that. Now, I'm not saying we still don't get down or scared, but I'm sure of one thing—when we sat around and did nothing, we both got depressed.

MARY: But there are times when I don't feel like doing anything. I just get tired. And I don't have anyone to pull me out of it.

JOE: That's all right. When you're tired, make sure you rest. Nobody's saying you have to go out and run the hundred-yard dash. If you don't get enough rest and take care of yourself, you can't expect to have the energy to do anything else. That comes first. As for having someone to help pull you out of it—I know that if I didn't find the energy within myself to do things, no one could make me do them. It has to come from inside you. Sure, it helps to have people to do things with, but it isn't necessary. And, Mary, what people are really saying is that, even if you can't do anything physically, do *something*. Do anything but sit around thinking about how bad you have it! That doesn't help.

MARY: But I can't help what I think.

BOB: Oh, yes, you can! If people couldn't control what they think, almost everybody with cancer would be depressed, and they're not. I think what people here are saying is that, even though they struggle with depression from time to time, they've worked out some strategies for dealing with it. One of the strategies is to keep busy. And the other is to look for positive ideas. I think what you are doing right now is good. You are here talking with all of us.

SAM: I'll tell you, Mary and Helen, I've got a fourteen-year-old boy with leukemia, and if you want to see how thinking differently changes things, you ought to see our family. My wife only looks at the bad things that might happen—and how bad they are right now—and she is literally a mess. I love her dearly, but she's a wreck. My son and I try to be hopeful as much as possible, and maybe we're not great, but we are making it. We're not naive. We're not hiding from the cancer. We know it's a tough disease and maybe he will die, but he's not dead yet. He taught me that. He's really been enjoying everything he can, even with his treatments taking so much out of him. So anything's possible.

SUE: Don't forget, like Bob said, we're with you. You've got us, with all our faults.

(All laugh a little.)

HELEN: I do appreciate that.

MARY: Me too. More than you know.

HELEN: I think you've given me some things to think about. I really am tired of being depressed. And maybe there's more that I can do about it. Some of you people sure have!

MARY: You know, I have a neighbor who's always suggesting I come for dinner or that we go shopping together. I've always put her off, thinking she really didn't want to do it. But I can see now that it was me who didn't want to. I think I'll take her up on her offer.

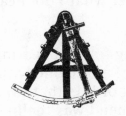

Guilt

ANN: Can I talk about something that's really bothering me?

SCOTT: Sure. What's going on, Ann?

ANN: My husband has Hodgkin's disease. We have a two-year-old baby girl. *(She takes a deep breath.)* I guess what's bothering me is that I feel really guilty about what is going on with me through this whole cancer situation.

SCOTT: What do you mean, Ann? Guilty about what?

ANN: Well, I think I should be spending most of my time worrying about Hank, but I'm not. I'm worrying about how we're going to pay the bills—we're having a tough time financially. I worry about what's going to happen to me and to the baby if Hank doesn't make it. Then I feel selfish and guilty. But I keep doing it.

SAM: Ann, I sure hope you don't think you're the only one who struggles with guilt! You're looking at a guilt expert here! I feel guilty because I can't do enough for my son. Then I feel guilty because I butt in to his medical program too much. Then I feel guilty because I'm not more help to my wife. And then I feel guilty because I get mad at her for being scared. No matter what I do, I can get myself into feeling guilty!

BOB: This is interesting for me, hearing about guilt from the family members' side. I'm the one with the cancer and I deal with a lot of guilt. Part of it is that I wish I had spent more time with my family when I was feeling well, instead of waiting until the cancer knocked me down. Now I have times, especially when I'm going through chemotherapy, when I'm pretty wiped out and I need a lot of help. I'm not used to having people do so much for me and I feel guilty about being a burden. To be honest with you, I never really thought about my family dealing with guilt.

SAM: I guess you're right. I didn't think about the guilt my son might have. Though, honestly, I'm not sure what it would be about. I'm not sure what I could do about it either.

SCOTT: What do you do with guilt? How do you handle it? Anybody?

LOU: Let me tell you what I did. It's not a hundred percent guaranteed, but it helps. When my wife got cancer at age forty-seven, I got angry. All the kids had just left home. We were getting ready to have a great retirement, and then wham! I really was mad at her for getting cancer. Then I felt really guilty. I thought, What kind of jerk am I, getting mad at somebody for being sick?

SAM: What did you do?

LOU: I told my wife, and she started to laugh because she was feeling guilty for being sick and messing up our plans. I jumped in and said, "Oh, don't feel guilty. That won't help anything." My wife looked at me and smiled and said, "I hope you were just listening to yourself, because you said some pretty good things about getting rid of guilt." She was right. When I started to help her with her guilt, I was helping myself. She still kids me about that. And we have had a wonderful retirement, in spite of her cancer. We made up our minds to do everything we wanted to do, and we worked around the disease.

HELEN: Maybe, in a weird way, I'm lucky. I was raised in a family who loved guilt. When I was in my late twenties, I said to myself, All this guilt stuff is getting me down—I can't move! So I quit feeling guilty.

ANN: Just like that?

HELEN: Well, sort of. I just thought, Who needs it? Guilt doesn't serve any purpose—it doesn't change anything. And if I really look at it, usually I feel guilty because I'm not living up to some super-high expectations for myself. Mine or someone else's. You know, superwoman, the perfect wife, the perfect mom. The perfect wife would think only of her husband, not about herself.

ANN: Yeah. That's me too.

HELEN: You can have that guilt junk if you want it. Not for me, thank you.

ANN: But what did you do? How did you get rid of it? I can't believe you can just quit feeling guilty!

HELEN: What really helped me was developing a sense of humor. You know, when you're feeling guilty about lots of things, it's usually because you're taking yourself just too seriously! You have to be able to keep your sense of humor. If you don't, you'll go crazy! Especially with cancer in the picture.

LOU: My wife and I decided we had enough sadness and tough times around without creating more for ourselves! When she starts feeling guilty about me doing things for her, I tell her that just by letting me help her she's doing something for me. That makes me feel good. And when I get tired and feel guilty about wanting a break, she calls her sister and tells me to take off for a while and get away. We both feel better.

ANN: It sounds as if you two have a wonderful relationship!

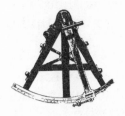

Embarrassment

JOE: We've been talking about opening up and communicating and all that stuff. I have something that's really hard to talk about—and that's a colostomy. You don't just say, "Hey, wanna see my bag?" or "Guess what I got today!" And I'll tell you what, even if I did want to talk about it, I'll bet nobody else would.

SUE: That's how I felt when I thought I had to have a mastectomy. But even with my scar, it's bad enough. Here I am, thirty-four, relatively pretty, and now what do I do? No man will want me. I was really into that kind of negative thinking. And you know what? Talking about it did help. I couldn't talk to my parents because they were still pretending I had an ingrown toenail or something like that, but the cancer support group really did help. Plus, a woman came to see me who'd had the same procedure done, and she showed me a lot and let me talk about my feelings. When you first hear you have cancer, you think only of whether you'll survive. After a while, though, you begin to have to deal with the ramifications of the treatment! Sexuality is such a big part of living normally, and when you have to adjust to something that makes you different—not only as a person, but sexually as well—it can really throw you for a loop!

BOB: You know, Joe, I think there's an organization of people who have ostomies. You might find them really helpful. The American Cancer Society could tell you where to find it.

SAM: Embarrassment is really tough to deal with. My son lost his hair because of the chemotherapy. It's come back now, but that was really hard on him. They told him it would happen, but it's one thing to hear about it and another to see big clumps of hair coming out of your head.

MARY: What did you do?

SAM: Well, first I asked him what he wanted to do.

SCOTT: I think that's really important. A lot of times we make decisions for others based on our own needs and feelings, even though they're not appropriate for the other person.

SAM: He said he wanted a wig. So we all went out together and tried to make it a fun experience. And, you know, it really was fun! We all got into trying on some outrageous wigs and laughed our heads off. Don't get me wrong, when the hair started coming out, it was traumatic for all of us, but at least we made the best of it. His hair is all back in now, and it's beautiful.

BOB: I guess my embarrassment involved my overall experience. I lost a lot of weight. I looked terrible. I went through a period when I wouldn't see anyone except my wife. Honest to God, I wasn't even letting my kids in. Of course, I said it was for their good, but I think I was just protecting my own ego.

SUE: You know, it's one thing to be a little embarrassed by the way you look, and I know that can be tough, but it's another thing to have...certain parts of your life potentially affected by the disease. I know sexuality is not an easy topic to discuss, but it's important. I'm still scared of being intimate with a man because of what happened to my body. I'm afraid he wouldn't find me attractive because I am a cancer patient and my body isn't perfect like you see in the movies. I think he would reject me.

HELEN: He wouldn't reject you if he loved you.

SUE: I don't mean he'd walk out and say good-bye, but that he'd see me as different.

JOE: Look, Susan, I don't mean to imply that you don't have a problem, but I'll bet you wouldn't trade it for this bag on your body. Now that isn't very attractive!

MARY: My husband had a bag on his body for fifteen years, and we still had a pretty good sex life, if I do say so myself!

HELEN *(laughing):* Well, good for you, Mary. It's nice to hear that spunk in your voice.

MARY: It was difficult at first because he was so aware of it all the time. But eventually it was no big thing. It's only a big thing if you make it one.

SUE: I know that in my head, but I'm still scared to tell men in my life about my illness. When I'm alone, it's easy to make sense of it. But when I'm with someone, I get uneasy. For instance, when do you tell someone? On your first date or what?

SCOTT: The real issue is how comfortable you are with yourself. If you're confident that you have a lot to offer someone, even if that doesn't include a perfect body, that confidence will shine through. A person who is really interested in you will only find you more interesting because you've had to deal with some real problems in your life.

BOB: I know that's true, Sue. You have a great deal to offer.

SUE: Thanks, everyone, for your support. It really helps.

ANN: Our sexual relationship sure hasn't been very good since Hank got sick. At first I could understand, because we were both scared and dealing with a lot of new things. Lately, though, he's been doing better, and there shouldn't be any physical reason for his lack of interest.

HELEN: Does he talk about it?

ANN: He just says that once he's—quote—cured—unquote, then he won't be preoccupied with getting well. We don't even hold each other anymore.

MARY: Sometimes it's good to talk to a counselor when you get stuck. It doesn't mean you're crazy, but that you need help.

ANN: I'm sure he wouldn't go.

SCOTT: Maybe a close friend could help out. It seems that people get all tied up inside about having cancer and doctor appointments. Constantly being prodded and poked and examined can really put your sexual self to sleep. It helps if someone works through that with you.

BOB: I think we pay more attention to the differences in ourselves than others do. We're often harder on ourselves than the people who care about us are, and that affects our relationships and our self-image.

SUE: I know that I'm at my best in dealing with the changes when I like myself. When I'm more insecure about myself, I focus on my body's imperfections and worry about what others think. I need to keep feeling good about who I am, not just what I look like.

LOU: You know, I think we're all doing pretty well. We each cope with things differently, and we each handle some things better than others. We can all learn from each other.

HELEN: I think if I ever get really afraid again—and I probably will—I'll think of all the ways you all have helped me by sharing your successes and your failures. I really have learned a lot.

BOB: Amen to that! We've all got a ways to go, but it's nice to know we are not alone. We have each other.

SCOTT: Maybe this is a good place to end this session. Thanks, everybody. And keep believing in yourselves!

About the Authors

Judith Garrett Garrison and Scott Sheperd have worked with hundreds of people with cancer and their families and friends, helping them see alternatives and discover new ways to help themselves. Through *Cancer and Hope: Charting a Survival Course,* they share with others the wisdom and courage of many who have undertaken this journey before them.

Judith Garrett Garrison, M.Ed., L.S.W.

In 1978, after giving birth to twins and with a three-year-old at home, Judy discovered she had lymphoma. Within weeks of that discovery, she was diagnosed as having dermatomyositis, another potentially fatal disease, which affects the immune system. Her physical condition deteriorated until she was bedridden, with a tracheostomy for breathing and a gastrostomy tube for feeding. Over a twelve month period, she underwent surgery, chemotherapy, and radiation therapy. During this difficult time, she made a commitment to help others going through similar experiences. She has kept that commitment.

In 1980, after her remarkable recovery, she proposed and was hired to implement a cancer support and education program at Flower Memorial Hospital, a regional cancer treatment center in Sylvania, Ohio, where she had received treatment. This program has evolved to include not only support and education, but media resources, training for health care professionals, and specialized volunteer services—all with the goal of assisting people coping with cancer. She has worked in oncology social work since 1981. In 1985 she became director of the hospital's social service department.

Scott Sheperd, Ph.D.

Scott Sheperd is director of the Institute for Training and Human Development at Flower Memorial Hospital. For over ten years, he has spent hundreds of hours working with people who suffer from life-threatening and/or chronic diseases—cancer, heart disease, diabetes, and others. His primary goal, whether in lectures or in individual or group counseling sessions, is to help motivate people to keep their physical disease from overcoming their spirit. He also works with professionals—physicians, nurses, and counselors—to help them be more effective in responding to patients' and family members' emotional needs.

Resources

Bolton, Robert. *People Skills: How to Assert Yourself, Listen to Others, Resolve Conflict.* Englewood Cliffs, N.J.: Prentice-Hall, 1979.

Bruning, Nancy. *Coping with Chemotherapy.* Garden City, N.Y.: Dial Press, Doubleday, 1985.

Bry, Adelaide, and M. Bair. *Visualization: Directing the Movies of Your Mind to Improve Your Health, Expand Your Mind, and Achieve Life Goals.* New York: Harper and Row, 1978.

Buscaglia, Leo. *Living, Loving, and Learning.* Thorobane, N.J.: Charles B. Slack, 1982.

Canton, Robert Chernin. *And Time to Live: Toward Emotional Well-Being during the Crisis of Cancer.* New York: Harper and Row, 1978.

Castaneda, Carlos. *Tales of Power.* New York: Simon and Schuster, 1974.

Cousins, Norman. *Anatomy of an Illness.* New York: W. W. Norton, 1979.

Davis, Martha, Elizabeth Eshelman and Matthew McKay. *The Relaxation and Stress Reduction Workbook.* 2nd ed. Oakland, Calif.: New Harbinger, 1982.

Fighting Cancer: Step by Step Guide to Helping Yourself. Kansas City, Mo.: Cancer Connection, 1985. (4410 Main St., Kansas City, Mo. 64111)

Fine, Judith. *Afraid to Ask: A Book for Families to Share about Cancer.* New York: Lothrop, Lee, and Shepard, 1986.

Fiore, Niel A. *The Road Back to Health.* New York: Bantam, 1984.

Freeman, Lucy, and Herbert S. Strean. *Guilt: Letting Go.* New York: John Wiley and Sons, 1986.

Graham, Jory. *In the Company of Others: Understanding the Human Needs of Cancer Patients.* New York: Harcourt Brace Jovanovich, 1982.

Haines, Gail K. *Cancer.* New York: Franklin Watts, 1980.

Hargrove, Anne C. *Getting Better: Conversations with Myself and Other Friends While Healing from Breast Cancer.* Minneapolis: CompCare Publishers, 1988.

Harper, Randy. *I Choose to Fight.* Englewood Cliffs, N.J.: Prentice-Hall, 1984.

Henry, Janet. *Surviving the Cure: A Time to Laugh.* Cleveland, Ohio: dist. by Cope, Inc., 1984.

Hutschnecker, Arnold. *Hope.* New York: G. P. Putnam's Sons, 1981.

Hyde, Margaret O. *Cancer in the Young: A Sense of Hope.* Philadelphia: Westminster, 1985.

Ireland, Jill. *Life Wish.* Boston: Little, Brown, 1987.

Johnson, David. *Reaching Out.* Englewood Cliffs, N.J.: Prentice-Hall, 1981.

Kelly, Orville. *Until Tomorrow Comes.* New York: Everest House, 1980.

Kushner, Harold S. *When Bad Things Happen to Good People.* New York: Schocken, 1981.

Larschan, Edward J. *The Diagnosis is Cancer.* Palo Alto, Calif.: Bull, 1986.

LeShan, Eda. *Learning to Say Goodbye: When a Parent Dies.* New York: Avon, 1976.

Levine, Stephen. *Meetings at the Edge.* New York: Anchor, 1984.

Morra, Marion, and Eve Potts. *Choices.* New York: Avon, 1980.

Pelletier, Kenneth. *Mind as Healer/Mind as Slayer.* New York: Delacorte Delta, 1977.

Pendleton, Edith. *Too Old to Cry, Too Young to Die.* Nashville, Tenn.: Thomas Nelson, 1980.

Ram Dass. *Grist for the Mill.* Santa Cruz, Calif.: Unity, 1977.

Rollin, Betty. *First You Cry.* New York: New American Library, 1976.

Rosenbaum, Ernest H. *Comprehensive Guide for Cancer Patients and Their Families.* Palo Alto, Calif.: Bull, 1980.

Shook, Robert. *Survivors Living with Cancer: Portraits of Twelve Inspiring People.* 1st ed. New York: Harper and Row, 1983.

Simonton, O. Carl, and Stephanie Simonton. *Getting Well Again.* New York: Bantam, 1980.

Simonton, Stephanie. *The Healing Family: the Simonton Approach for Families Facing Illness.* New York: Bantam, 1984.

Sontag, Susan. *Illness as Metaphor.* New York: Farrar, Straus, and Giroux, 1978.

Spingarn, Natalie. *Hanging in There.* New York: Stein and Day, 1982.

Thomas, Frank P. *How to Write the Story of Your Life.* Cincinnati: Writer's Digest, 1984.

Trull, Patti. *On with My Life.* New York: G. P. Putnam's Sons, 1983.

Waller, Sharon. *Child of Hope: A Child Rescued by Love from a Medical Death Sentence.* New York: Bell, 1983.

Weisman, Avery D. *Coping with Cancer.* New York: McGraw-Hill, 1979.